SHUT
UP
AND
RUN

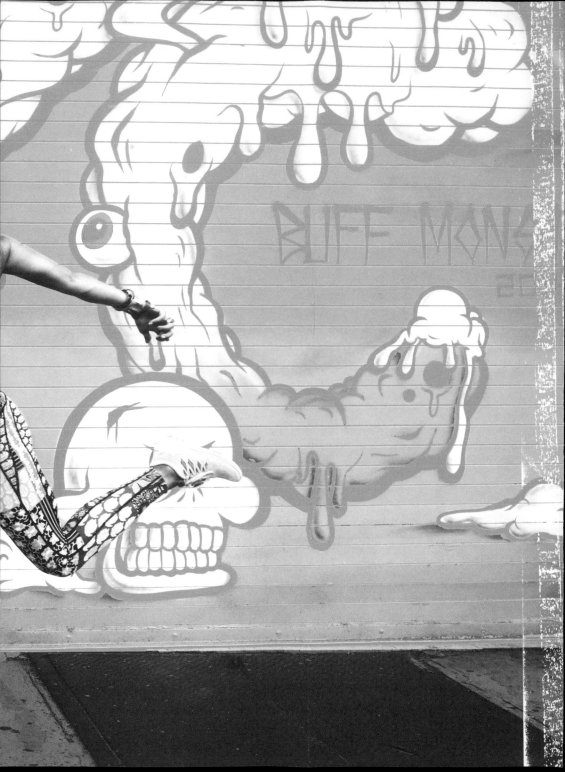

SHUT
UP
AND
RUN

HOW TO GET UP, LACE UP, AND SWEAT WITH SWAGGER

ROBIN ARZÓN

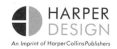

HARPER
DESIGN

An Imprint of HarperCollins Publishers

HarperCollins books may be purchased for educational, business, or sales promotional use. For information please e-mail the Special Markets Department at SPsales@harpercollins.com.

First published in 2016 by
Harper Design
An Imprint of HarperCollins*Publishers*
195 Broadway
New York, NY 10007
Tel: (212) 207-7000
Fax: (855) 746-6023
harperdesign@harpercollins.com
www.hc.com

Distributed throughout the world by
HarperCollins*Publishers*
195 Broadway
New York, NY 10007

ISBN 978-0-06-244568-1
Library of Congress Control Number: 2015945533

Book design by Stislow Design

Printed in the U.S.
Third printing, 2017

The information in this book has been carefully researched, and all efforts have been made to ensure accuracy. The author and the publisher assume no responsibility for any injuries suffered or damages or losses incurred during or as a result of following the exercise program in this book. All of the procedures, poses, and postures should be carefully studied and clearly understood before attempting them at home. Always consult your physician or qualified medical professional before beginning this or any exercise program.

DEDICATED TO MY MOM.

TO THE REBEL.

TO THE SQUARE PEG IN THE
ROUND HOLE.

THIS BOOK IS ALSO FOR YOU,
DEAR READER,
AND TO EVERYONE
WEARING AN INVISIBLE CROWN.

CONTENTS

"COME, COME,
WHOEVER YOU ARE.
WANDERER,
WORSHIPPER,
LOVER OF LEAVING—
IT DOESN'T MATTER.
OURS IS NOT A
CARAVAN
OF DESPAIR.
COME,
EVEN IF YOU HAVE
BROKEN YOUR VOW
A HUNDRED TIMES,
COME, COME AGAIN,
COME."

—RUMI

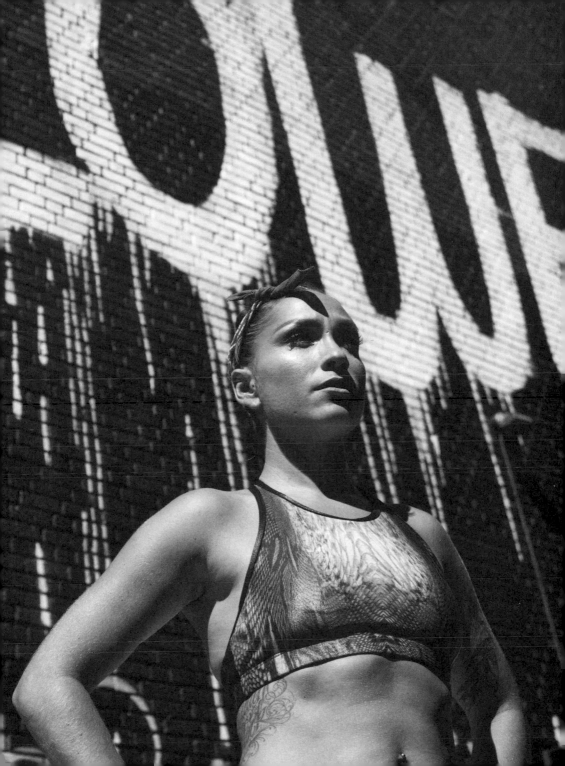

INTRODUCTION

"ANYTHING THAT GETS YOUR BLOOD RACING IS PROBABLY WORTH DOING."
—HUNTER S. THOMPSON

"SHUT UP AND RUN."

THIS WAS THE MANTRA I USED to endure the hours until I could leave my desk as an eighty-hour-a-week New York City litigator and lace up my running shoes. I ran my first mile at age twenty-three in between studying contract law and criminal procedure. Fast-forward seven years, to when I'd find myself running five marathons in five days across the mountains and deserts of Utah, thinking, How the hell did I get here?

Running shoes were instruments in my liberation. I became absorbed in the drumbeat, the cadence, of my footsteps. Twilight runs beckoned me to get lost in the motion, only to discover myself. Eventually, these miles gave birth to my Tumblr blog, SHUT UP & RUN, in 2010, and soon I found myself running right out of a law career to sweat with swagger and move with abandonment. I decided to do one thing with my life—epic shit—and I want you to come along for the ride.

As a running coach, ultramarathoner, and journalist, I became part of a world of urban athletes who don't just run—they live to move on their own terms. We push the pulse of cities with our feet. We don't "jog," or count calories, or give a shit about high school 400-meter track records. We are a living mash-up of culture, sport, fashion, and storytelling. *Shut Up and Run* is about running as a lifestyle. It's where fashion meets sport. It's how we tell stories through movement and feel good while doing it.

Part fitness collective and training platform, *Shut Up and Run* provides tips, tricks, and visual motivation on how to cultivate moments of sweat, laughter, miles, swagger, friendship, and authenticity. *Shut Up and Run* is a resource unshackled by self-doubt and from which ordinary people can learn to do extraordinary things; it provides a platform for running, jumping, twerking, and working in the way only endorphins can.

This book is a compendium of inspiration that makes you want to move and is rooted in information that shows you how. What's my mission? To redefine what it

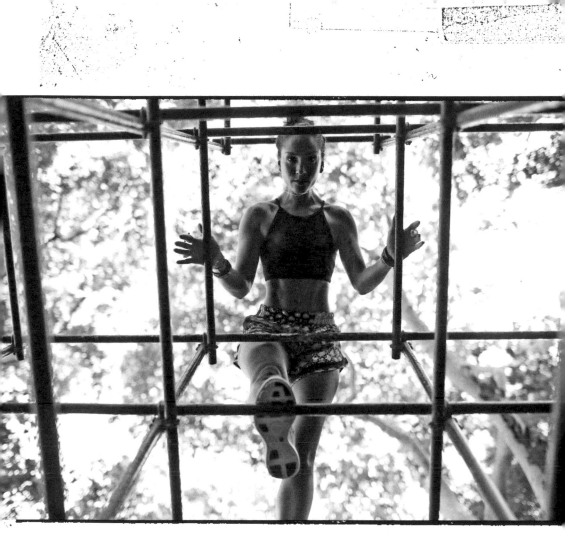

means to be an athlete and create unapologetic greatness in every athlete along the way. This book is a platform to do the things that make us go "Damn!" when we're one hundred. It's a daring adventure of athletics and style.

Let's unlock passion through movement, mindfulness, and by doing epic shit. My lessons from a life lived in sweat are laden with nothing but possibility for you to do it, too. What do I want people to know about running? It's actually not that complicated.

Welcome to *Shut Up and Run*, where you'll discover how to test the limits of your potential. All you need is a heavy dose of swagger and a pair of running shoes. The revolution will be delicious. Can you taste it?

"BAND-AIDS DON'T FIX BULLET HOLES."
—TAYLOR SWIFT, "BAD BLOOD"

WHAT IF you found yourself in a situation where you had to be braver than you ever imagined you could be? At the age of twenty-one, I discovered just how brave I could be when an evening that started with me catching up with old friends ended with a gun to my head.

Approaching my senior year at New York University, I was just off work from my summer job as a legal assistant at the law firm Querrey & Harrow and planned to meet up with my college roommate Mel and her boyfriend Ryoji. We stumbled upon a small wine bar in the East Village called Bar Veloce. None of us had heard of it before—this was presmartphone era, when Yelp reviews allow you to experience a place before you've actually been there—but it looked like a good spot to grab a drink.

We found open seats at the bar and ordered drinks. As we were sipping our wine, a man walked in, a well-dressed guy who muttered, "I've been shot."

I turned to Mel and said, "Is this a joke?"

In 2002, reality television was gaining traction and I recall thinking this was a terrible, tacky TV stunt.

Next entered a man who I would later learn was named Steven Johnson. He shot the man in the doorway, who then fell to the floor.

In that moment, time slowed. I'm certain the writers of *The Matrix* must have experienced this type of trauma. Remember the scenes where Neo is slowly falling backward, almost touching the ground in an epic backbend, and then stands upright? Yeah, it was that kind of slow.

Johnson immediately came at me. As he yanked me back by my hair, all I could think was, He's so strong for being so skinny. The feeling of hair being ripped out of my head was a new sensation, but in a situation like that you don't feel pain as you tumble over chairs and get jostled in the mayhem sparked by a man with a gun. At least I didn't.

"Motherfuckers are leaving in body bags!" Johnson yelled.

And I believed him.

You know the movie *Sliding Doors* with Gwyneth Paltrow? I've always been mesmerized by the thought that one turn, one choice, can change your life. That night, there were two choices, two directions to take. You could either go straight, which led to the kitchen and a dead end, or left, which led to freedom on Tenth Street via the bathroom window. Ryoji and Mel ran to the back of the bar and turned left. Dragged by my hair, I was led to the kitchen.

There were twenty hostages and one angry guy with three pistols and a samurai sword. He threw me on the ground.

The swinging doors to the kitchen were two hundred feet from the front entrance. The narrow aisle gave us a line of sight to the busy Manhattan evening happening outside. I could see police cars had arrived, but freedom seemed far. Standing in the swinging doors, Johnson shot toward the street. An old Asian man looked in the bar to inquire about the commotion. Johnson shot him, too.

"Tie people up," Johnson demanded, throwing plastic zip ties at me.

I remember the focus in this moment being similar to the way Michael Jordan describes making a basket in a basketball game—time slows and the hoop becomes as large as the moon. I did what I was told, the mental wheels in my head turning frantically, but staying surprisingly on track.

Maybe if I make this loose enough people can get out, I thought to myself as I tied up some of the hostages.

Suddenly, I felt liquid being poured on my head. It burned the cut on my scalp where my hair had been ripped out. I recognized the smell and saw a long red barbecue lighter appear in Johnson's hand. He flicked sparks in people's faces as he poured more kerosene over us.

"Motherfuckers are leaving in gasoline shirts today."

I realized then that this wasn't a robbery. He wanted people to die, and I was one of those people. He grabbed me firmly by the back of the neck and drew me in front of him like a human shield. The only things I was aware of were a gun pressed to my right temple, a barbecue lighter to my left, and my beige, urine-soaked slacks.

I still remember the outfit I was wearing, a throwback to my lawyer days when I scoured Ann Taylor or Loft for discounted suits with some semblance of personality. When I left the office that day clad in a sleeveless, silk shell shirt and beige pants, I could never have predicted I would lose bodily functions in them as a result of horror and fear.

I could see the NYPD officers outside from where I stood.

"You're going to be all right," Johnson murmured in my ear.

Suddenly I feared a new threat. RAPE. As my brain tried to sort through the madness in search of meaning, I shed not a single tear. I distinctly recall dry eyes and an alarming sense of composure when he addressed me directly, personally, intimately.

"What do you want?" I asked, realizing, maybe for the first time, that this was very fucking real.

"I want to talk to the police outside!" he screamed, more expletives flying.

If saliva were flammable, his words would have singed. His anger was palpable, but his reasoning was lost. As I grabbed my Nokia cell phone from my pocket to connect with the police outside, I assumed a role I was wholly untrained to do: negotiator.

"Nine-one-one, this is Robin Arzón. I'm at Bar Veloce on Eleventh Street. There's a man with a gun, Steven Johnson, and he wants to speak to the NYPD officers standing outside."

I handed the phone to Johnson, who proceeded to demand that the cops outside close the front door to the restaurant.

I summoned the courage to ask, "What do you want from these people here? You have control, but what is it you want?"

"I want them to close the fucking door. Motherfuckers are leaving in body bags!" he bellowed.

The officers, in head-to-toe black gear, wielding shields and rifles, looked like they were out of a Tom Cruise movie. I had nothing but cinematic references in my cortex. None of this made sense in my lived experience except for what I had witnessed in other people's fiction. Somehow fiction was becoming my reality and I had the barrel of the gun pressed against my head to prove it.

In the moments that followed, our exchange became personal.

"You'll be okay," he said. "Yo te entiendo," he continued in Spanish.

He speaks Spanish. I can personalize this somehow. If I humanize this then maybe he'll be less inclined to shoot me in the head. I had never been more grateful that my Cuban mother and Puerto Rican family imparted their native tongue to me.

"Entiendo. Y que quieres? Tienes gente aqui con familias que aman."

The police asked that he release the hostages, at least the women. He spun us around, looking at the huddled hostages behind, and retorted, "I only see white women in here. White people are going to die."

The clarity with which one acts under this type of duress reminds me of those stories you hear of the mother who lifts a vehicle to save her infant pinned beneath. I wanted to try to calm him down. We talked in detail about his family, his son, his wife, who had recently died. The moments when he spoke about his family were his most intelligible. Those were also the pauses when all I could hear was the voice inside myself screaming with ache and rage that this would not be the end of my story.

The end of this narrative would come from the bravery of a stranger, Ann-Margret Gidley, a blond twenty-something woman with blue eyes and full lips. She was sitting in the wash basin in the kitchen five feet behind us, slightly more elevated then the rest of the hostages, and had a direct line of sight to Steven Johnson and

THE HUMAN BODY
IS CAPABLE OF
EXTRAORDINARY
THINGS THAT ALL
START WITH THE
CHOICE TO TRY.

myself, the human shield. She noticed him struggling while attempting to hold me, the gun, the cell phone, and the barbecue light. When he holstered the gun in his waistband, she jumped at him from the basin.

I felt a falling sensation and hands around my neck. I heard a gunshot. And then another. The hands were so tight around my neck I was thinking, If he's been shot, how is he still so strong? And then I was free from his grasp.

Ann-Margret had tackled him to the ground. The bravery of this woman single-handedly saved everyone in Bar Veloce that night. The bold microdecisions we make have impact.

I saw a NYPD officer standing above me. I still don't know his name, but the sight of his gentle eyes is something I'll never forget. As quickly as it started, it was over. I was sitting outside the bar where my life almost ended, now being interviewed by police officers.

You don't need to come close to death to be reborn if you remember that you're made for more. Surviving that awful night became the catalyst for my catharsis. I picked up a pair of running shoes as an escape from living through that hell. Running became my liberation from pain, fear, and anger.

SWEAT WITH SWAGGER

EVERYTHING IS A MIXTAPE. The conversations and creations of our generation are a remix of things that preceded us. I'm talking about real OGs—"original gangsters"—like Plato, Aristotle, and Socrates. We're having an existential moment that has come before, and will come again, where inspiration abounds, "mindfulness" is a common dinner topic, and sweat can equal happiness. Given the luxury of understanding the value of time, we're constantly thinking of how best to spend it, record it, and capture it, and what those snapshots say about us to the world.

From the bards traveling from town to town retelling Homer's *Odyssey* to linear prose during the rise of the Enlightenment, storytelling holds no truer or more fragmented space than it does now. The omnipresent idea of "newness" through the stream of visual conversations on social media put the magnifying glass to our own stories. "FOMO" (fear of missing out) and "YOLO" (you only live once) are colloquial references to now. Our prison is the voice inside our heads that says, "no, won't, can't."

At a certain point, we begin to tell ourselves stories, to define what we "are." Most of us live under the dominion of how the world defines us—what our job says about who we are, what our past says. Those statements not only precede us, but silently lead us into unconscious shackles of other people's standards.

Shut Up and Run is about taking back your story. Using fear as fuel, together, let's ask questions, disrupt destructive paradigms of self-loathing, and accomplish things that make others go, "Damn . . ."

"Swagger" might be common jargon now, but let's not confuse the situation. Swagger is earned. It can be grimy or graceful. It can be innate, but it's also finessed. It's the feeling that makes you sit a little taller and reinforces your backbone. We sweat with swagger when we infuse a shameless confidence into movement. To sweat with swagger is to redefine what it means to be an athlete and create unapologetic greatness along the way. When we sweat with swagger, we test the limits of human potential. When our footsteps are powered by motivation and a strong community, the cadence is a drumbeat to doing something epic. Sweat is magic. Swagger is the glisten.

Thanks for coming on this journey to *Shut Up and Run.* I know a lot about running. I don't know everything. This is not my memoir, your full training guide, or an encyclopedic take on endurance sports. This book is meant to be a resource, a fun place for inspiration and information. I'll always keep it real and give you my opinion. Feel free to disagree with me. I can take it.

Also, I curse a lot. Let's play.

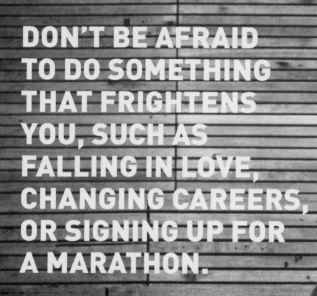

DON'T BE AFRAID
TO DO SOMETHING
THAT FRIGHTENS
YOU, SUCH AS
FALLING IN LOVE,
CHANGING CAREERS,
OR SIGNING UP FOR
A MARATHON.

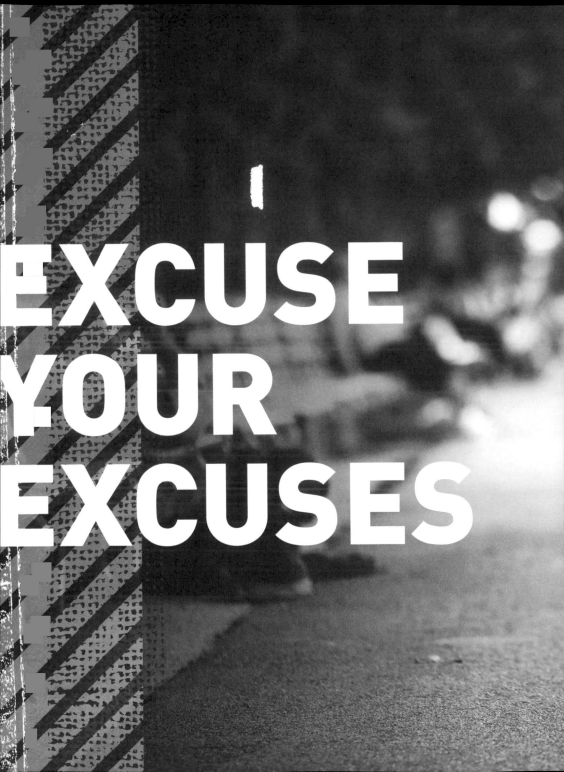

EXCUSE
YOUR
EXCUSES

REGRET IS
A HEAVIER
WEIGHT TO
CARRY THAN
HARD WORK—
IN RUNNING,
LOVE, AND
LIFE.

Before we start, I want to be clear with what I'm all about and where I've come from.

I've never won a race and I don't run a five-minute mile, though I have major respect for people who have done both (check out my list of running superheroes on page 184).

Growing up in the suburbs of Philadelphia, I didn't play a single sport. I was the arts-and-crafts kid. As my cousins competed in soccer and track, I watched from the sidelines telling myself I was not an athlete. Fear created my content, not my dreams. I defined myself by the story I was telling myself.

However, I re-created myself, and so can you. After years of making excuses, in 2012 I decided to quit my career as a corporate litigator at Paul Hastings LLP and booked a ticket to London to write about the Olympic Games as a freelance reporter for my blog and publications like *Newsweek* and the *Daily Beast*. Since then, I've run thousands of miles and completed 50- and 100-milers. Most important, I love this shit. I love the sweat. I relish the moment when "can't" becomes "can." The endorphins we gain from running cannot be bought at Whole Foods or a juice shop. The confidence that running unlocks comes with a high that is earned, not given. I know that life. I'm about that life. I want to share it with you and I want you to share yours with me.

BEGIN ANYWHERE.

START
BEFORE
YOU'RE
READY.

TODAY
SEEMS
LIKE A
GOOD
DAY.

WHAT'S YOUR STORY?

"I'M A RUNNER."

Often, thinking those three words is harder than taking the first physical step to being one. I didn't run my first mile until I was twenty-three and it took thousands of miles before I owned this part of my story. I want you to own your narrative from the first block, mile, or kilometer, because if you're putting in the work, you deserve the title RUNNER.

Toeing the line of my first 10K, I was surrounded by "real runners." They may as well have been unicorns—the elusive athletes wearing the perfect gear, moving effortlessly, at a pace I couldn't fathom. By projecting my insecurities on them, I became "other." I was the outsider encroaching in this special space that was the racecourse, the track, the street, or even the treadmill.

I call bullshit.

The funny thing about stories, namely, our own stories, is that they are largely composed of irrational thoughts we tell ourselves. Sometimes you just have to fake it till you make it. So lace up, puff out your chest, and just go for it. It's the act of moving one foot in front of the other that makes you a runner, not the little voice in your head uttering, "no," "can't," "won't." Flipping that story can be tough. This chapter is all about channeling the voice inside that writes our story. Our inner monologue can turn *can't* into *can* and dreams into realities. Extinguish doubt with action. Let's write the story that says we are a little better than yesterday. We can push ourselves to where we want to be. It's going to take a little sweat, though. Happy is something you do, baby, and only *you* are responsible for your happiness. Life is happening right now, so stop making up excuses and tell me, what do you want your story to be? Do you want to be a runner? Have you always dreamed of completing a marathon? Whatever it is, write it down, look back on it, and own it.

TIPS FOR WRITING YOUR STORY

Appreciate the struggle. The path to success is circuitous. Enjoy the journey. There might be a lot of pain before that runner's high becomes your jam. Not every run will be your fastest, most exciting, most endorphin-filled session. That's okay. Believe in yourself.

WRITE YOUR STORY

_____

_____

_____

_____

_____

_____

_____

_____

_____

_____

_____

_____

_____

2. Write your story using fear as fuel.
Does it get your blood pumping? Does it make you nervous or scared? Then that's a challenge you were meant to encounter and tackle. Own the pen to the story you're writing. Let the discomfort of the thoughts in your head saying "no" guide you to "yes."

3 Pay attention to the little voice inside.
Dr. Fred Luskin from Stanford University estimates that people have more than sixty thousand thoughts a day and most are repetitive. This means our inner monologue is on repeat. Begin to listen to what it is saying. Ignore the self-doubt and skepticism, and listen to the little voice inside that says you can be faster, stronger, and better.

4 Use your superheroes as motivation.
Write down your superheroes. This could be your mom, She-Ra, Serena Williams—anyone you admire and respect. The point of this exercise is to motivate yourself and to remind you that even champions started at zero. Every single one of them had to deal with struggles and own their narrative. If their story inspires you, how are you going to pay it forward?

SUPERHERO TOOL KIT

Here are some essentials that will get you going. There's a *ton of shit* out there being sold to runners. Don't get overwhelmed. Start out with a good pair of running shoes. We'll go through all the extra fun stuff you can buy in Chapter 7.

1. **Shoes:** Go to a local running store and get fitted for shoes. The fly ones might not be good for your feet, so choose wisely and don't be afraid to ask for help. I strongly recommend getting a gait analysis so that you get the right shoes for your feet.

2. **Headphones:** I don't run with music much anymore, but I totally get that jams keep you moving. Some good headphones for active folks are Monster iSport Bluetooth Wireless, Yurbuds, and Jaybird X2 Wireless, because they are made to withstand bouncing and sweat.

3. **Sports bra and shorts:** In the beginning, feel free to wear whatever you have in your closet so long as its comfortable, doesn't cause chaffing, and, for sports bras, offers support. Your dope running wardrobe will come.

4. **Water:** My rule is if you're planning to run forty-five minutes or more you want to be sure to have water accessible to you, either from drinking fountains along the trail or carried on your person. For runs that are forty minutes or less, hydrating before and after the run should be sufficient, so long as it's not blazing hot outside.

5. **Inspiration page:** Start a running log, keep a notebook, or make a mood board to get yourself inspired. It also helps to follow social media accounts that make you happy and get you motivated to get out there and run.

6. **ID:** Run with your driver's license in case of an emergency. I also recommend investing in a Road ID bracelet.

7. **Running watch or GPS app:** These range from twenty dollars to hundreds. Unless you're training for an Ironman or need crazy metrics and data, a free app such as the Nike+ Running or Strava is good in the beginning to measure your pace and distance.

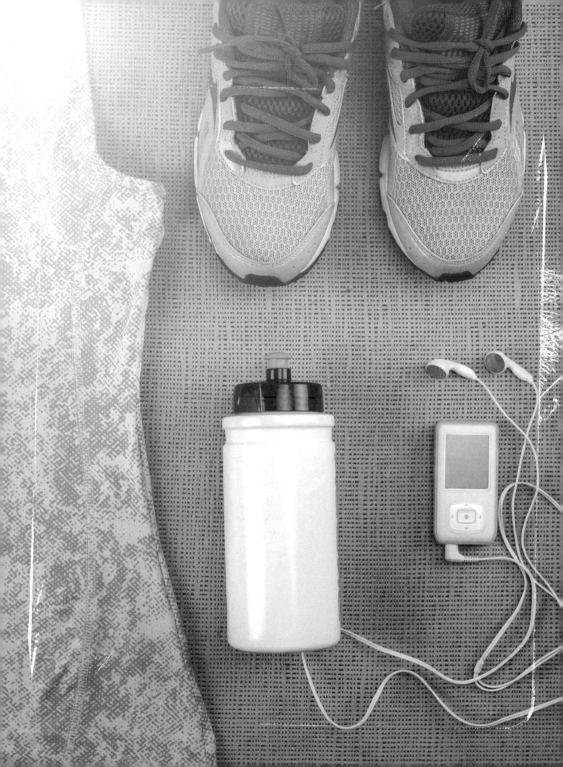

COMMUNITY BREEDS ACTION

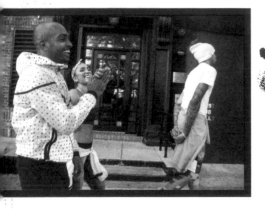

THE JOURNEY OF THE SOLO RUNNER is well documented. The racecourse, your training, your finish line, all depend on one person . . . you. However, my running world exploded when I started training with the NYC BridgeRunners, a motley group of runners in downtown New York City who meet weekly to make the city their racecourse. No rules, just great vibes, running, and sweat. The miles I've logged with the BridgeRunners unlocked parts of my potential I didn't know were there. They offer the encouragement and motivation that come with running shoulder-to-shoulder, stride for stride, with a homie.

Even though running is inherently a solitary sport, and even if you enjoy solo runs, I strongly recommend trying a local group run. Street athletes are everywhere. You can ask your local running store if they host weekly or monthly runs. If not, start your own. If you ask them, they will come. People just need a reason. Meetup.com is also a great site to find active folks in your area, or you can join mapmyrun.com or Strava and train virtually with fellow runners. Start a hashtag campaign to track your progress and stay accountable. You can also sign up for a race and talk to someone else doing the race, too. The point is to find your fellow weirdos. Not every run will be with them, but the memories of the miles will fuel you for a long time to come.

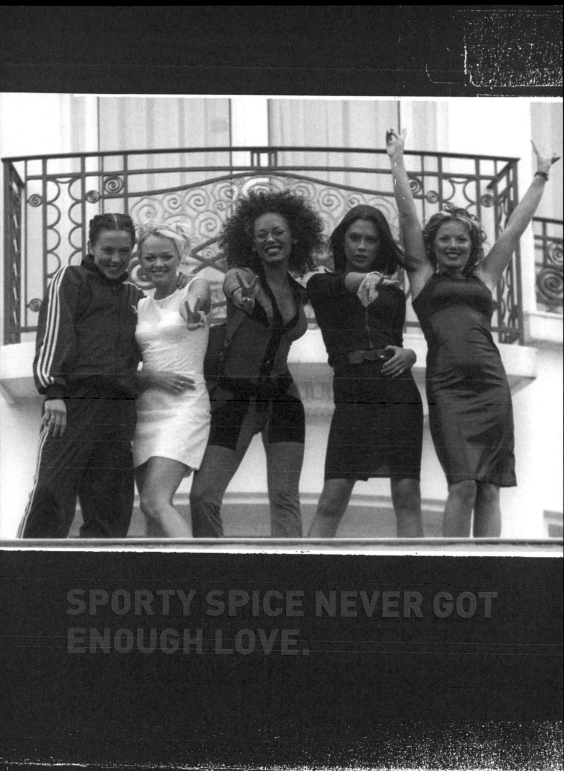

SPORTY SPICE NEVER GOT ENOUGH LOVE.

REASONS TO GET OFF YOUR ASS

THERE ARE MANY WAYS life, weather, excuses, or the voice in our head tries to roadblock us. Those days when you don't want to run. At all. Excuse your excuses!

SEVEN TIPS FOR GETTING OFF YOUR ASS WHEN YOU REALLY JUST WANT TO WATCH NETFLIX

1. Get fly gear. If you look good you will feel good and want to move.

2. Go for a run while listening to 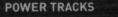 (Beyoncé, duh!)

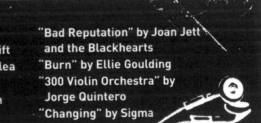

POWER TRACKS

"Upgrade U" by Beyoncé
"Shake It Off" by Taylor Swift
"Heavy Crown" by Iggy Azalea
"Thursty" by Bassnectar
"Till I Collapse" by Eminem
"Slam" by Onyx

"Bad Reputation" by Joan Jett and the Blackhearts
"Burn" by Ellie Goulding
"300 Violin Orchestra" by Jorge Quintero
"Changing" by Sigma

3. Think about the possible regret you'll feel for skipping, compared to the mad endorphin high you'll get from running.

4. Get out the door and just do ten minutes. If you need to stop, stop. But once you've started, I bet you'll finish.

5. Keep your earbuds fresh with new SoundCloud jams or an audiobook. I often listen to Eckhart Tolle's *The Power of Now* or the Rich Roll podcast during tough runs.

6. Surround yourself with inspiration. "Do epic shit" is written on a Post-it on my bathroom mirror *and* it is the title on my alarm alerts on my iPhone.

7. Remember why you started. Identify the "why," and the "how" will follow. Some days you really just need to rest and watch TV. That's cool. But that's not every day, baby. Choose wisely.

VISUALIZATION TIP

Conjure a memory of a time when you felt like you were on top of the world.

I MEAN IT.

One moment—no matter how long ago or what the circumstances were—when you felt invincible. Write it down below in detail. How did you feel? What were you wearing? Who was there? What was the weather? What did the air smell like? These are powerful memories we can draw on when we need a little boost. Our bodies can react to the memory when we viscerally relive the confidence and power from that moment. Can't think of one? Create one. Dream really big.

LOVE YOURSELF TODAY AS MUCH AS KANYE LOVES HIMSELF. THAT'S A LOT.

YOU
ARE
HERE

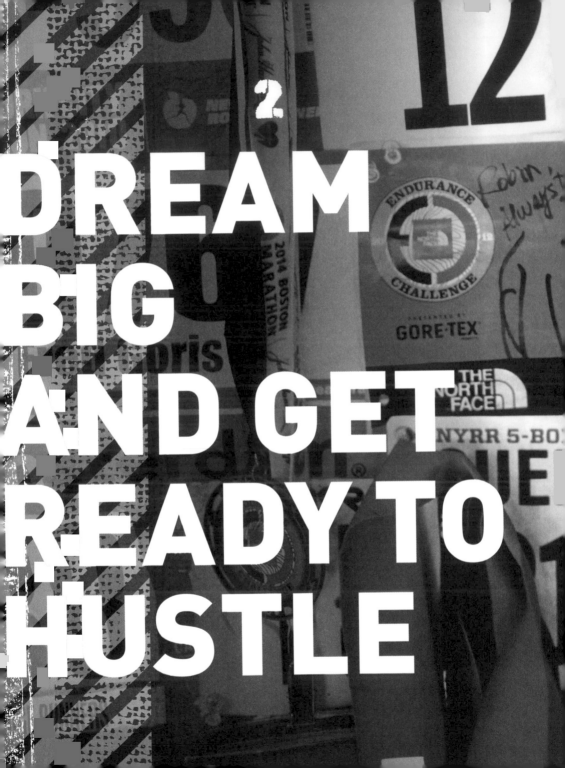

EVERY DAY IS
A CHANCE TO
BE GREAT.
WHY NOT TODAY?

MY FIRST RACE EVER

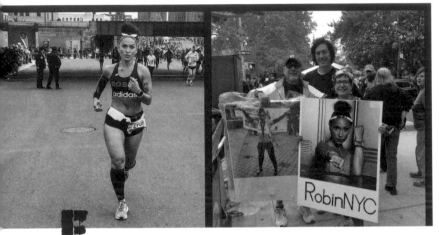

FOLLOWING THE INCIDENT AT BAR VELOCE, I spent the next year finishing up at New York University, in talk therapy, and mostly in focusing on being happy. I was alive. The magnitude of living has never been lost on me from the moment the gun touched my temple.

IF YOU ARE BREATHING, IT'S A GOOD DAY TO HAVE A GOOD DAY.

My running life started before I put one foot in front of the other. I was figuratively running from my own thoughts after being held hostage. The barrel of a gun pressed against your temple is something you don't forget. The smell of kerosene and the feeling of helplessness would creep up on me while I was waiting for the subway, making tea, or setting my alarm for work the next morning. I buried these memories, the anger and pain of trauma, by distraction—going out, working, TV, drinking. I was distancing myself from the patterns that controlled my mind by staying busy. I didn't want to think, so I worked. I started law school at Villanova University the following fall. That's when I laced up and ran it out.

One day, on a break in between Torts and Contracts, I saw a flyer for a 10K starting and ending the following day at the Philadelphia Museum of Art. I didn't have a smartphone and it didn't occur to me to google how far a 10K was in miles. On an impulse, I decided to sign up for it. Like a moth to a flame, I found the pull to run to be strong. Only now when I reflect on that first 10K do I see it was the weight of trauma that propelled me to move. I see it was the catharsis, but in the moment it was just one other crazy thing I would add to a list of other arbitrary crazy things I'd eventually do, like surfing with sharks off South Africa or canyon jumping in Switzerland (by the way, I highly recommend both).

I showed up at seven the next morning in sneakers that hurt my feet and wore the shirt they gave when I signed up at the race table that morning. (FYI: Don't do that. You look like a tool). I ran that day. I ran the entire 6.2 miles without stopping, but not without cursing and questioning why running was so hard after all those hours I'd spent at 2.0 speed on the elliptical.

Crossing the finish line I vowed one thing: that *that* distance would never feel that hard again. Through running I was able to unlock parts of myself that I didn't know were there and let go of the shit that was weighing me down. And I didn't stop.

I fell so in love with it that I kept running after I graduated from law school and moved back to New York City. Running in the city unearthed an entire world. Every run felt like an exploration. Each corner felt like a microcosm of adventure. I stumbled upon the NYC BridgeRunners running crew and I was home. I found a tribe of people for whom running was a lifestyle and sweating with swagger was an ethos. I started running with them religiously every Wednesday night, no matter what excuse I had to give to get out of work in time or how late I had to work after the run concluded. My Tumblr blog, SHUT UP & RUN, was born after I signed up for my first marathon, the New York City Marathon, in 2010. I wanted to do just that—shut up and run through the city I loved. I had no idea then just how many miles in New York I would run and that my hobby, the run, would become my most important relationship.

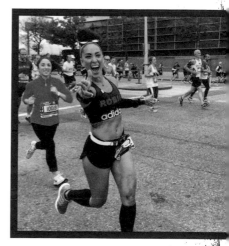

THE RUNNER'S MANIFESTO

WEAK IS NOT IN THE ITINERARY.

We are a boundless movement calling for sweat.

We are proof that every day you can walk out and change your life.

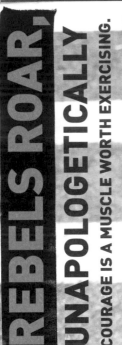

REBELS ROAR, UNAPOLOGETICALLY.

COURAGE IS A MUSCLE WORTH EXERCISING.

TO DO:
SWEAT.
BURN.
REPEAT.
Train
for
life.

WARRIOR

isn't just a yoga pose, it's a state of mind.

MAKE THEM LOOK TWICE.

TRADE SWEAT FOR STRENGTH.
SWAP DREAMS FOR PLANS.
LEAP FEARLESSLY.
YOUR FUTURE SELF IS WAITING.

LOSE EXCUSES; FIND RESULTS.

**START UNKNOWN. FINISH UNFORGETTABLE.
GRIND, WHILE OTHERS MAKE EXCUSES.**

GOODBYE, "I wish . . ."
HELLO, "I will!"

SILENCE
YOUR INNER HATER.
DON'T STOP UNTIL
YOU'RE PROUD.

YOU SHOULD COLOR OUTSIDE THE LINES.

THIS
IS
YOUR
ROAD
TO A
FINISH
LINE.

WELCOME
TO A
FAMILY
forged in
sweat.

**SHUT UP
AND RUN!**

RUNNERS' CHEAT SHEET

IN THE BEGINNING OF MY RUNNING CAREER, even perusing an issue of *Runner's World* sent me into anxiety mode. The things I now geek out over (aka the latest issue of *Runner's World*) used to make me feel overwhelmed. If you're prone to WebMD'ing and going down the Internet rabbit hole stalking training plans, tips, tricks, shortcuts, etc., then *step away* from the computer.

Running is awesome because it's accessible. You can do it anywhere and you don't need a lot of fancy gear. Here are some beginners' running tips to get you started. It's not that complicated. You've got this.

1. **Get the right shoes:** I cannot stress enough the importance of purchasing good running shoes. I saw someone running in Jordans, which might look iconic on the basketball court but are not made for distance running. I get the dedication, but stop. As I mentioned earlier, go to a local running store where they can observe your running form and recommend shoes for your gait. And, no, they might not be the hottest new Nike Flyknits, but it's important that you run in what's right for your feet to avoid injury.

2. **Listen to your body:** I'm all about pushing your limits, but listen to your body so you can tell when you need to pull back. There's impending injury and then there's being a wuss. If you start to feel muscle aches, then stop, stretch, and get back into it slowly.

3. **The talk test:** A lot of runners go out of the gate too quickly, get winded, frustrated, and swear off running. Slow. It. Down. The next time you go out, try the "talk test." If you can sing a verse from your favorite song or have a conversation without panting, then you're at the right pace. You've got to learn to jog before you sprint, ya feel me?

4. **The 10 Percent Rule:** Increase your cumulative mileage no more than 10 percent a week. In the beginning, once you get in a running groove, you might want to go headfirst into crazy miles. DON'T! Abide by the 10 Percent Rule. Slow and steady increases will keep you progressing and injury free.

5. **Don't stress about the miles:** I recommend starting out clocking your runs by minutes, not miles. Begin at fifteen minutes, twenty, twenty-five, and build from there. Once you're comfortable running for thirty to forty minutes, then you can start tracking miles, either using a smartphone app (such as Nike+ Running), MapMyRun.com, or any GPS-enabled device. Run on feeling, not on numbers.

WHAT'S YOUR RUNNING GOAL?

FOR NEW RUNNERS, starting out can be challenging, but it's all about being willing to get uncomfortable. Step out of your comfort zone. That's when change happens. You have to get to the top of the hill before you can really see the view.

Best way to keep going? Holler. Tell someone about your goal to start running. Post it on Facebook or Instagram, or start a blog about your journey. Call your mama. Why? Because putting it out there keeps you accountable. Do what you said you would, and let those inspired by your actions sing your praises. What you do matters.

Set realistic goals, but set them. Identify the "why," and the "how" will follow. Commit to a realistic goal like three runs per week for one month, or sign up for a 5K (check out www.active.com), and then tell someone about it. Better yet, get them to join you!

Remember: you are a runner. What is a "real" runner? You. If you're putting in the time to sweat and get moving, you are a runner. I don't care how fast or slow you are, or how many runs you've done. Create yourself and never apologize.

Starting out can be hard. I know the feeling. You're new. You're slower. You apologize.

"Sorry, I'm totally gonna hold you back."

"Sorry, this is my first race."

"Sorry, I just don't know if I can do this."

I'm calling bullshit on these apologies and here's why: you are amazing for taking one step. Even experienced runners were novices once. Every runner, even Olympians, remembers needlessly apologizing. It's one thing to acknowledge and respect someone else's pace, training plans, and your perceived limits. That's respect. It's another to apologize for existing, for newness, for weight, for awkwardness. Own it all. And when you don't feel like you can, pick up this book and fake it until you make it.

CHALLENGE: Identify one running goal you can accomplish this week, such as running your first mile, mapping your longest run, signing up for a race, or getting your first pair of running shoes. Write it down and tell someone who will keep you accountable. You have seven days to do this. Your excuses are excused. Remember, if it makes you nervous, even better. Go!

BE OPEN TO
GETTING LOST
SO THAT
YOU END UP
MOVING IN
THE RIGHT
DIRECTION.

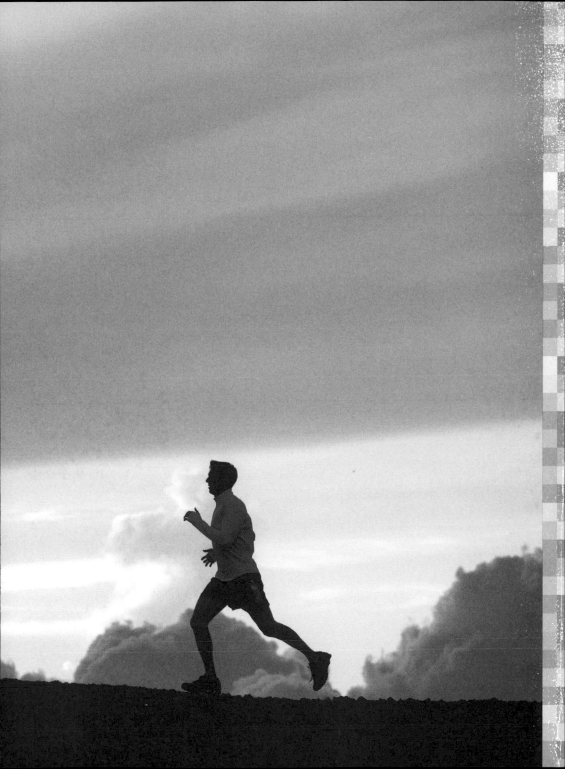

"TO GIVE
ANYTHING
LESS THAN
YOUR BEST
IS TO
SACRIFICE
THE GIFT."
—STEVE PREFONTAINE,
AMERICAN RUNNER

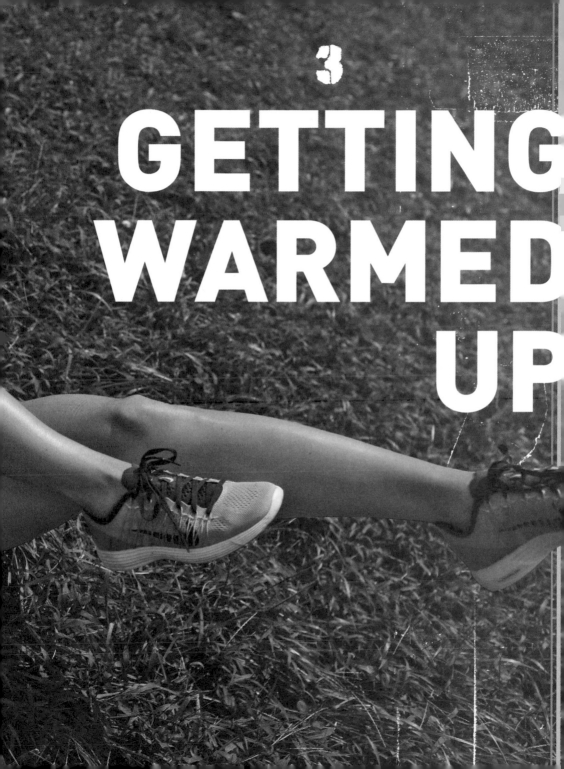

3

GETTING WARMED UP

RUNNING THROUGH HEARTBREAK:
My First New York City Half Marathon

LOVE MAY MAKE THE WORLD GO 'ROUND, but heartbreak fuels risky behavior. And I support it. When Britney Spears released "Womanizer" and Beyoncé belted "Run the World (Girls)," centuries of heartbroken women responded with two snaps and a head swerve. Uh huh, honey. We've all been there.

Ross and I were the perfect, dynamic couple, until we weren't. We dated for two years and our breakup in March 2010, the same week of my first NYC Half Marathon, sent me into a hole so deep that I thought my heart would calcify. Although it's been nearly ten years since we first met, we're still friends. Energy doesn't lie. However, in that moment the pain was cavernous and the sadness was palpable.

I had been running roughly twenty miles a week, mostly alone and without direction. In fact, I had been training for my first half marathon with Ross planning to cheer me on, only for our breakup to happen the week prior to race day. Instead of Ross, I had family along the racecourse as I took to the streets of Manhattan determined to run the entire 13.1 miles. Heartbreak lit a fire under me so hot I was engulfed in flames. And I did it. With that earned medal around my neck, I went home and signed up to run a 26.2-mile marathon the following November with the New York chapter of the National MS Society.

The next six months of training changed my life and helped me get over Ross. Not only did I discover my body could cover vast distances, but I was also welcomed by a running community that helped to heal me. From the New York City BridgeRunners, my running home, to the Jackrabbit NYC Marathon Training Program, led by Coach Jonathan Cane, I became me again.

Remember in *Waiting to Exhale* when Angela Bassett's character gets the sway back in her hips and the light back in her smile after her divorce proceedings? Well, running is how I got my groove back and you don't have to be dealing with loss to appreciate the transformation. In fact, I hope you don't. But if you've been there then you know. Sweat heals.

Now, for the most important question of this book: why do you run? If you identify the "why" then the "how" will follow. Why are you lacing up? Trying to get faster? Trying to get over heartbreak? Aiming for a personal record (PR)? Gunning for your first mile? Our reasons will change, but if you can clearly name them it will be harder to fall off course. I signed up for my first marathon to get over a breakup.

My "why" was heartbreak. That made getting up at 6 a.m. to run, longer than I had ever contemplated, possible because I needed to run it out. The reasons can and should change as your life and running coalesce, as you progress, and the universe speaks through movement. Your reason might be longevity, waist size, community, sex appeal, vanity, pride, love, curiosity—as long as it's *your* reason, it's valid. Own it. Marinate in it. And remind yourself of the WHY when you're searching for a HOW.

TODAY
IS THE
DAY

TO BECOME
YOUR OWN
INSPIRATION.

HOW I GOT MY GROOVE BACK:
Ten Tips for Getting Started

TRAINING FOR MY FIRST MARATHON FOLLOWING MY BREAKUP, mile after mile, I healed. And in the cheesiest, most *Eat, Pray, Love* way possible, I crossed that finish line in Central Park a different version of myself, a better version. When you feel the weight of the medal around your neck, after powering through the city you love, blowing kisses to family at mile 21, you feel like a damn warrior. I still draw on that moment when doubt creeps in.

Running is a lifestyle, a marathon is a journey, and each race opens up a different part of you. It all starts with a single step.

1. A walk/run program is not lame. Do whatever it takes to get off the couch, even if that might involve eating a piece of humble pie. Be honest about how your body is feeling and where your fitness level is right now. This is especially important for former athletes and those coming off a long hiatus. You will get it back, but start small.

2. Discomfort is normal. You must get used to some discomfort and soreness, but sharp and debilitating pain is not the name of the running game. If you're not sure about the pain, try to walk for a minute or two to see if it disappears. If something lingers and feels wrong then stop and consult a specialist.

3. Feeling breathless is normal, but gasping for air is not. Slow down if you can't hold a conversation. Breathe through your nose and your mouth.

4. Cramps and side stitches are common for new runners because the core muscles aren't used to it. They will go away as your fitness level increases. When you get one, breathe in deeply and stretch out your diaphragm around your rib cage. Lift your hands above your head, relaxing your shoulders, and stretch with a slight upward motion.

5. When you're identifying running routes, look for a route that has even footing and is well lit. The quaint area with cobblestone paths or a dark trail is not the best place for running.

6. If you're going for a run under thirty minutes you don't need a ton of shit. Carry water if you feel like you absolutely need it, but there's no need to eat a huge

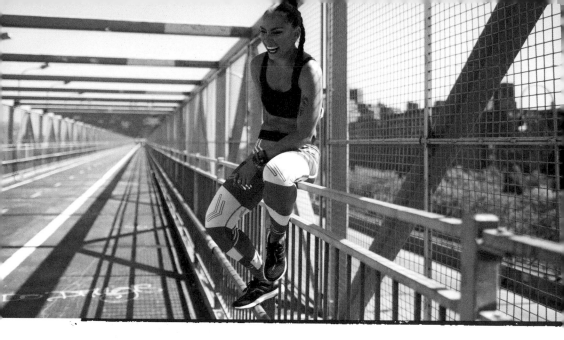

meal or load up on gear. Keep the run simple. You. Running shoes. Clothes. That's it.

7. You will fail. There will be days when you hype yourself up to go for a run and you just don't make it out the door. Try again tomorrow. What matters is that you don't stop trying to get it done. That said, try to find a time and stick to it. Habit goes a long way in creating consistency.

8. Don't try looking awesome yet. This is new and you're not supposed to look like someone on ESPN. Concentrate on how you feel.

9. Opt for cheap technology. The time may come when you invest in a sick GPS device to measure your runs. There are seriously impressive watches out there, but you don't need one in the beginning.

10. Get a physical. You want to make sure you're okay to run, and a physical is also a great way to gauge basic numbers for head-to-toe health. Just as you will track your runs and, eventually, your miles, it's smart to know your blood pressure, resting heart rate, cholesterol level, and general fitness level.

CHALLENGE: I want you to go on a run for minutes, not miles. That means no watch or app tracking your distance. This first venture might be ten minutes or thirty. Just run until you get tired. What matters most during these first few sessions are the gradual change to your muscle memory and, most of all, the confidence to know that you laced up and got out.

RUNNING SMART AND SETTING GOALS

BALANCING PATIENCE AND DRIVE IS KEY because results take time. Bite-size goals that provide incremental progress allow us to celebrate little victories instead of feeling guilty when we miss overly ambitious goals. It's absolutely possible to train from the couch to a marathon. I've seen it done many times. However, you need to understand the time commitment to training and the lifestyle changes that come with it.

Focus on one or two clear goals. If you were driving a car across the country you would plan a route, places to stop, and a game plan, right? This is no different.

BITE-SIZE GOAL SETTING

- Create a mission statement, both short term (three months) and long term (one year or more) from now. What *exactly* do you want to accomplish?

- Think SMART (a goal-setting acronym that stands for Specific, Measurable, Attainable, Realistic, and Timely). "Getting fit" is not as helpful as "mastering inversions in yoga" or "going to kickboxing twice a week for four weeks." By what magnitude do you want to get stronger, faster, happier? How much weight do you want to lose and by when?

- Establish a baseline. Take a before photo. Clock that next run. Set an intention for *each* workout. One goal to reach. One reason you're pushing for it. Track your progress. Number crunching might seem horrific, so use technology to help. Food journals. Running apps. There's something for you.

- What is your *passion*? Let it lead you. It can come from anywhere, but it has to be yours. If you establish the "why," the "how" will follow. If the hot guy who checks you in at the gym is your motivation for showing up, so be it! Think about what excites you. If you've always wanted to slaughter a mud run, think about the specific workouts and steps that will get you there. Passion drives progress.

- Tell someone. Your friend, your boss, Facebook. It helps keep you accountable, allows people to encourage you, and might connect you with others who have similar goals. POST IT. Make it known.

- Make calendar appointments. Think about a past success to get yourself up. Do you function better in the morning? Do you work better as part of a team? Remove the obstacles. Lay out your clothes the night before or join the gym that's on your way home.

Screw New Year's resolutions that you know you're not going to keep. Instead, step up to being the CEO of your *body* for 365 days, little by little. Being the strongest version of yourself is the ultimate lifetime resolution.

PROGRESS IS NOT LINEAR. IT'S CIRCUITOUS.

CELEBRATE TINY VICTORIES.

WARMING UP BEFORE A RUN

- Jog/walk for five minutes. Going all out from the first step is asking for injury. Start out walking or lightly jogging to warm up your muscles and get the blood pumping.

- Striders are a common way to incorporate speed work, improve form, and warm up. Striders are flexible and involve speeding up your pace for 20–30 seconds and then slowing back down. The effect of picking up the pace will increase your stride length and foot turnover. After a few minutes of jogging accelerate your pace for 100 meters (or a block) and then resume jogging pace.

- Do dynamic stretches. Static stretching is when you hold a muscle in one position intending to elongate it; it is generally discouraged before a run because static stretching cools your muscles down when the goal is to warm them up. However, dynamic stretches can improve mobility and loosen muscles. Examples of dynamic stretches are butt kicks, side shuffles, squats, leg swings, and toy soldiers (walk forward lifting one leg at a time and touch your toes with the opposite hand). You want to do about five minutes of dynamic stretches before any run. They will warm up your muscles without taxing your body.

RUNNING FORM

Running economy will make you faster. However, even some of the most famous runners in the world didn't have perfect form. Long-distance runner Paula Radcliffe famously runs with an awkward gait and she's the fastest female marathoner to date. That said, there are mistakes that might cause injury and definitely don't contribute to efficiency. I'm culpable of all of them at some point or another. Here they are:

- Crossing your midline with your arm swing, or the center of your chest where your sternum is, wastes energy. Keep the angle of your elbows at 90 degrees with your hands in front of you, maintaining that same position in the back-swing when your elbows graze your rib cage. I recommend sitting in front of a mirror to practice.

- Hunched shoulders and bad posture happen when we are tired and/or have minimal core strength. Focus on fixing both with core work and a head-to-toe body scan during training runs—raise your shoulders to your ears a few times during the run and intentionally relax them down. The forward lean that occurs during sprinting and propels forward momentum starts from the ankles, not from an awkwardly slouched torso, ya dig?

- Clenching your fists stunts your stride. Pretend you are holding a potato chip in each palm and keep the pressure light enough that you wouldn't crush it.

- Overstriding happens when you aim to go faster or farther by taking a longer stride. This results in hitting the ground harder, usually on your heel, and no increase in speed. To avoid this, focus on swinging your arms faster and increasing your turnover (the rate with which each foot hits the ground). Your legs should do what your arms do, meaning you are one body of motion and a stunted arm swing will make for an awkward gait, and vice versa. Ideally, your foot should make contact with the ground while underneath your body. Olympian Jack Daniels dubbed 180 steps per minute as the ideal running cadence and that's pretty much the standard.

- Heel striking gets a bad rap because your foot hits the ground twice, once at the heel and again at the forefoot, instead of just in the mid- or forefoot. I get it. But some people are just heel strikers. I don't think I've ever run a marathon without resorting to heel striking when my legs are tired. There are always ways to tweak your form for safety and efficiency. A mid- or forefoot strike might reduce impact and increase efficiency, but I don't think there's anything inherently dangerous about heel striking. Think about how your body is moving as a whole. If something feels off, then it's probably worth adjusting.

- Running too slowly will negatively affect your form. A great way to build the muscle memory of what it feels like to have good form is to sprint on the track. Focus on your arm swing, your turnover, cadence (your rhythm), controlled breath, engaged abdominals, relaxed shoulders, and a forward lean, where your body is in a front-facing motion starting from the ankles to the top of the head. I find these come together most frequently for folks when they are sprinting.

Ultimately, if you've been running for a while and haven't had any injuries then you're probably running just fine. There's no sense in making your form worse by changing it just because of the latest study on arm swing, stance time, and all the other technical bullshit.

FINDING YOUR PACE

If you've been racing for a while, then you already know your pace for certain distances and likely have goal paces for specific PRs (personal records). If not, you will in due time. You want to establish a pace for as far as the race distance. Your goal is having the ability to increase your race pace for speed work and reduce it for recovery. The baseline—or your race pace—is created by you and will change on any given day or season as you progress, fall off, come back, and recover.

Your easy pace can be determined by the "talk test" mentioned earlier. If you can continue a conversation then your pace is chill. If you feel like you're panting a lot, then slow down. Of course, if the goal is a tempo run or a sprint and you can still belt "I Will Survive" you might want to pick it up.

Take it to the track and run one mile. Warm up by jogging for 5–10 minutes, then set a timer and go for it. Most tracks are 400 meters for one loop and 4 laps for a mile (1,600 meters). You don't have to go all out, but push harder than you normally would for a longer distance. This is likely your "push" pace. Repeat this once a month during training to see your progress. This can also be a good marker for the bulk of your training miles, which should be thirty seconds to two minutes slower than your track miles.

A running watch is an obvious tool to determine pace. Again, running apps are a less expensive option, and I still recommend taking the time to intuitively feel a pace by relying less on gadgets and your measured distance, and more on feeling and perceived exertion.

CROSS-TRAINING

I believe every single runner should cross-train. I'm a cyclist as well as a professional indoor cycling coach. I know cycling has improved my VO_2 max (maximal oxygen consumption), leg turnover, and overall cardiovascular fitness. Strength work, specifically body weight work like push-ups, squats, and TRX suspension training, is key to becoming an all-around athlete and a more powerful runner.

Of course, balance is also key. I know too many bucket list marathoners who expect to maintain their routine of yoga and spin and only run once a week. No. I also know the other extreme—runners who can't do a single push-up. Don't be either of those people.

YOU'RE THE CEO OF YOUR BODY. THE BOSS DOESN'T CANCEL.

RECOMMENDED SPORTS

Spinning pushes you aerobically and anaerobically without impact. In classes, like the ones I teach for Peloton, you work high-intensity intervals to build oxygen intake as well as tackle monster hills. Riding at a cadence similar to your outdoor running cadence (80–100 beats per minute) will maintain or improve leg turnover. Of course, actually getting outside on a bike can achieve this, too; it just takes more gear and more time.

Yoga keeps your muscles limber and gives you an internal sense of balance. Ease into yoga practice once a week well before any big race. It's not simply sitting there and breathing, it's building up muscle strength. You will work and create space in places you didn't know existed.

Rowing is a no-impact, high-intensity cardio. It is also a wonderful option for runners coming off leg injuries. Go to a studio that teaches classes and have someone show you proper technique.

Swimming is another winner for those coming off an injury. As a technical sport, it can help runners work on muscle weaknesses they were unaware of. The breathing capacity of swimmers astounds me. Who couldn't use that?

Strength exercises are also important and I recommend every runner learn how to do a proper push-up, plank, and squat. There are a million ways to get stronger, but those three moves are the base of your strength pyramid. Any trainer or boot camp class instructor can show you how to perform one properly. There's also YouTube, which offers countless videos on technique.

WHEN YOU
LACE UP,
ANSWER THE
QUESTION,
"WHO AM I GOING
TO BE TODAY?"

CHASE A DREAM.
CATCH A BETTER VERSION OF YOURSELF.
WHAT IF WE PRACTICED COURAGE
EVERY SINGLE DAY?
WHAT IF WE HELPED EACH OTHER
EXTINGUISH DOUBT—MILE BY MILE?
26.2 REASONS TO TRUST *YOUR* STRUGGLE.
BECAUSE OUTSIDE YOUR DOOR THE WORLD IS WAITING.

RUN THIS TOWN. RUN YOUR TOWN.

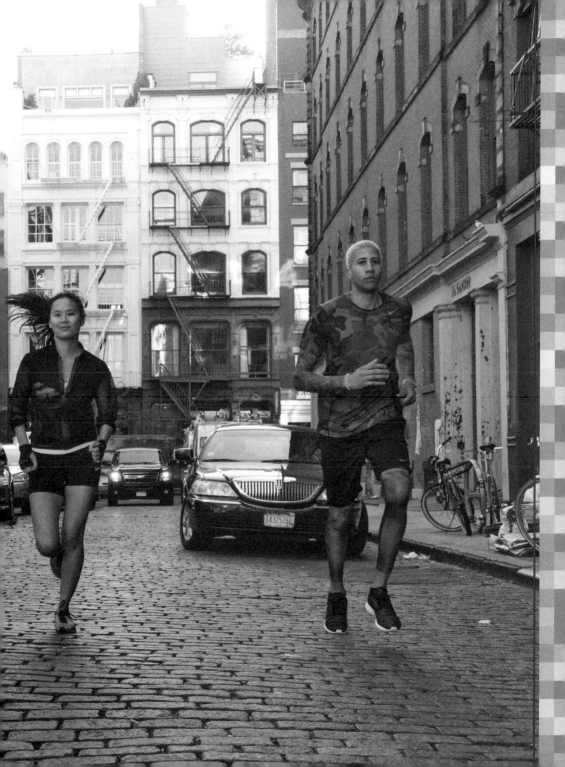

DEALING WITH A RUNNING WIDOW

YOU'RE GETTING INTO A RUNNING GROOVE. Running has become your jam. You don't understand why you haven't been doing this your whole life! Guess who might not be as excited? Your partner, friends, and family who don't run and cannot fathom your excitement over this new, sweaty obsession.

The running widow is real, people. When you're logging hours of miles a week, especially for endurance races like marathons and ultras, it's a lot of time away from home, and your friends and family may feel like they lost you to your hobby.

I've been lucky to date guys who also run and completely understand my level of

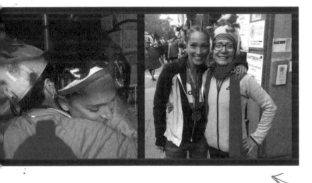

insanity. It's almost a prerequisite for me because I don't want to hear shit about going for a four-hour run whenever I need to, but I understand that's not the reality for some. My family has also been very supportive and they've been into it from day one. My mom has been to more races than I can count wearing this crazy hat. How lucky am I?

IF YOUR TRIBE ISN'T SO JAZZED ABOUT YOUR RUNNING, HERE'S HOW TO DEAL WITH IT

1. **A happier you is a happier them.** Communicate how running makes you feel and how that will make you a better parent, sibling, spouse, or friend.

2. **Invite them to join.** Maybe you can't get them to run, but take a recovery day and ask them to go for a walk with you. You can also have them bike alongside you, or ask them to meet you for lunch after a long run. Sometimes people just want to be asked to be included, even if they don't actually want to participate. I get that running may be "your thing," and that's okay. But once in a while extend the invitation.

3. **Don't expect them to cheer you on at every race.** When your elderly relative asks if you "won" your latest race with more than fifty thousand participants, just smile.

4. **Explain to them how they can best support you.** I dated a guy once who traveled with me to a 50-miler across the country. I was shocked when he didn't immediately provide the exact prerace silence and postrace soothing that I needed. How the hell was he supposed to know? Do you want a big party after you complete a race or solo time? Do you want signs along the course? Specific snacks? Tell them.

5. **Show them the support you expect in return.** Does your partner love golf? Book them a tee time. Do they relish a movie marathon? Set a date for one during your taper before the race.

6. **If you're running ultramarathons,** consider carefully who you ask to serve on your crew along the course. Emotions can get intense while running an ultra and you need someone who isn't going to take this personally! Ultra runners, myself included, can vacillate from superheroes to toddlers in a matter of miles.

7. **Not everyone will get your passion to run.** The honest truth is you might catch some shade. It's not about you! The criticism is really about them and their insecurities. You're one of one. Proceed accordingly.

VISUALIZATION TIP

ON RACE DAY, BEFORE YOU START, I WANT YOU TO VISUALIZE THE COURSE. This requires doing your homework beforehand and checking out the course. If you can't run parts of the course during training, then look at the elevation changes and mile markers online. That Fifth Avenue incline during the New York City Marathon will be a lot easier to tackle when you know about it in advance. Some racecourse videos are available online. Check the race site or YouTube for course information and imagery of landmarks. Note any landmarks that will serve as visual motivation. Mentally flag the aid stations. Take yourself through the course step by step and "run" yourself through potentially tough parts like hills and dead zones without crowd support.

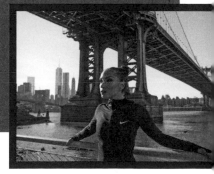

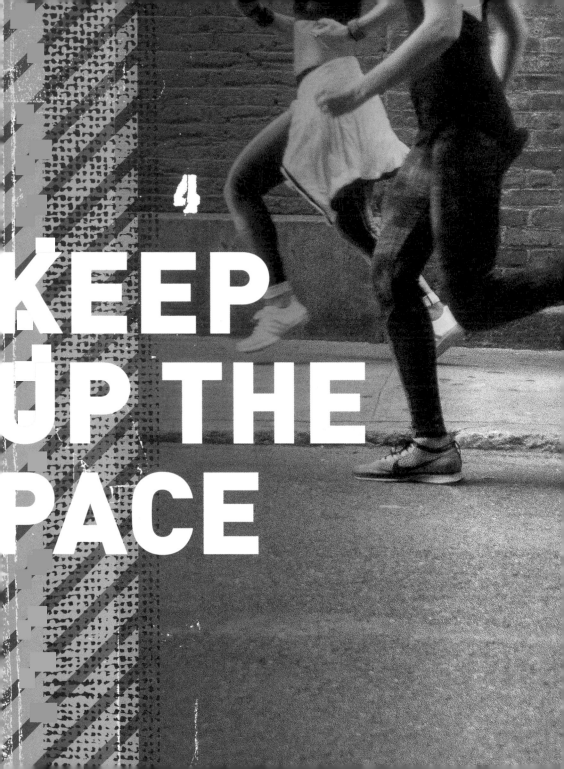

4

KEEP UP THE PACE

LIVING AT
FULL THROTTLE
TAKES HARD
WORK AND
SACRIFICE.

You work upwards of sixty hours a week. You pride yourself on keeping up with your juggling act of work, home, family, and self. You like to sweat and claim finish lines, but you don't always have time to train, so you cram it in on Saturday and Sunday.

Hello, weekend warriors. I know your kind. I used to be you. This chapter is dedicated to tips for staying in shape on the go and how to be efficient with your runs.

MY LIFE AS A LAWYER . . . AND THEN NOT

AS A CORPORATE LITIGATOR at Paul Hastings, I worked eighty-hour weeks. I ordered a ton of Seamless food deliveries, took summer associates out to two-hour lunches, and worked my ass off for some really smart people and impressive clients. I also counted down the hours until I could run, spin, or train with my personal trainer. It didn't take long before I realized I was leading a double life—the Robin who practiced law 80 percent of the time and the Robin who lived passionately as an athlete the remaining 20 percent.

I make no illusions that the transition happened over night or that it's realistic for you to do the same. There was no one singular *Jerry Maguire* moment during which I threw papers around my office and slammed the door to my old life. My firm was flexible enough to grant me a five-month leave of absence for me to travel and pursue running opportunities with companies like Nike in the United States and Europe.

After I had a taste, I couldn't look back. Leaving a six-figure, stable income was terrifying. It felt like I was jumping off a cliff, but in my gut I knew I could marry my skill set of writing, oral advocacy, and client engagement with a new career.

While visiting the NikeLab 1948 store in London, I happened upon the CEO of Nike Inc., Mark Parker, who has mythic status as one of the most innovative business minds in the world. Widely known as a gracious leader, he's also a former marathoner (he ran the Western States 100!) and a bona fide sneaker head, having started at Nike as a footwear designer more than twenty years ago.

Since I was working with the brand as a freelancer at the time, I went to introduce myself. Parker quietly pointed out some of his designs found at the store that are still strongholds decades later. We chatted about my recent departure from law in pursuit of my running passion.

"I considered going to law school," Parker remarked, "but then I took a job at Nike designing shoes and here we are."

Clad in all-black Nike Frees, Parker exuded a tangible passion for the brand—a brand that effectively encapsulates energy in motion and propels the world's most elite athletes. Parker complimented the American flag scarf wrapped around my head and my Air Jordan 1 jacket, a vintage find from around the time Parker started at Nike.

"You should start a fashion blog," he said.

The details from here are a bit fuzzy because I couldn't actually believe I'd just received the greatest compliment of my life. Today Parker probably doesn't remember our meeting, but that ten-minute interaction somehow legitimized the free fall that was this new, scary career change to freelance journalism. Standing before greatness, I handed Parker my business card with butterflies in my stomach before we parted with a handshake and a nod. Who knows if I will ever get the chance to thank him for the inspiration, but the stars aligned at the right moment to remind me that with big risk there's big reward. I still had no idea what the hell I was doing. I fumbled and made a million mistakes, but I was curious, hungry, willing to learn, and my own best advocate, even (especially) when I was bullshitting.

What the career would be was the question. When I left the field of law, I initially told people that I was a journalist. I had every intention of freelancing for fitness magazines for about five minutes but realized two things: 1) it pays one-eighteenth of my rent; and 2) nobody knew who the hell I was or would give me writing gigs. I had to reassess my game plan and create my own boxes. When you live in predetermined categories it's a lot harder to rise.

People often ask me what to do if they're unhappy in their career and want to change. That is a subject for another book, but, I will say this: make an honest assessment of how you want to feel at work every day. I believe this will inform what you want to do, at least in part. Also take note of people who you're jealous of because this will shed light on things you crave. Dissect those feelings of jealously to illuminate what it is about that person's gig that makes it desirable.

Once you have a career target (or five; who says it should be just one?), do an honest, gut analysis of what skills you have and what skills you need. You might need to make sacrifices, learn new stuff, and go back to school. You will, without question, have to knock on doors, ask for favors, do more work than you're paid for, and question your sanity all the time. Guess what makes it worth it? The hustle, baby. It's worth the work to live your dream. Regret is a heavier weight than hard work in your career, love life, and, sure as hell, in running.

RUN COMMUTE

RUNNING TO OR FROM WORK is the number-one way weekend warriors can sneak in extra miles without disrupting an already packed schedule. What about a change of clothes and arriving at work sweaty? What will coworkers think? There will always be excuses. I get it. You just have to decide how badly you want it. Ultimately, commuting to work is badass and chances are your boss will think so, too. There are worse things to be known for than as the person who runs.

Here's how I did it. I had my dry cleaning delivered to my office, so I had fresh suits. I told my coworkers about this new run commute plan and arrived early enough so that most didn't see me anyway. I joined a gym close to my office so I could shower nearby. Two words: baby wipes. Chances are, unless you live in a really hot climate you don't need to shower after every single run. Baby wipes, deodorant, dry shampoo, and baby powder go a long way.

COMMUTE TO WORK TIPS

1. **Plan ahead.** Pack work clothes the night before. To avoid bringing clothes every day, bring several outfits on Monday so you're set for the week.

2. **Keep spare socks and underwear in your office.** These are often forgotten!

3. **Have snacks and breakfast on deck.** Make a game plan for food once you arrive at work. Maybe you run with it or maybe you have an oatmeal stash in the office pantry.

4. **If you're commuting predawn,** it will be dark and I recommend investing in a headlamp. Stay safe.

5. **Leave time to freshen up and stop sweating.** If your office doesn't have a shower, look into a local gym, pool, or community center with a locker room. If the nearest gym is still too far, again, I strongly recommend using baby wipes, baby powder, and dry shampoo.

6. **Investing in the right running pack is essential.** I have used the same Camel-Bak pack for years. I take the water bladder out most of the time when I need

to carry more gear. For women who have a smaller upper body, look for packs made for narrow shoulders to avoid chafing.

7. **Run home after work instead.** This is a great option if you don't want to deal with showering at work, packing clothes, or having coworkers see you dripping in sweat. The caveat here: some workdays go long and enthusiasm can wane when your couch is calling.

8. **Play with distance.** If your direct commute is too long a run, see what public transportation options are available at the desired distance from the office.

9. **Keep a set of toiletries at work.** If you don't have a desk or a locker, ask maintenance if you can stash some items in the cleaning closet.

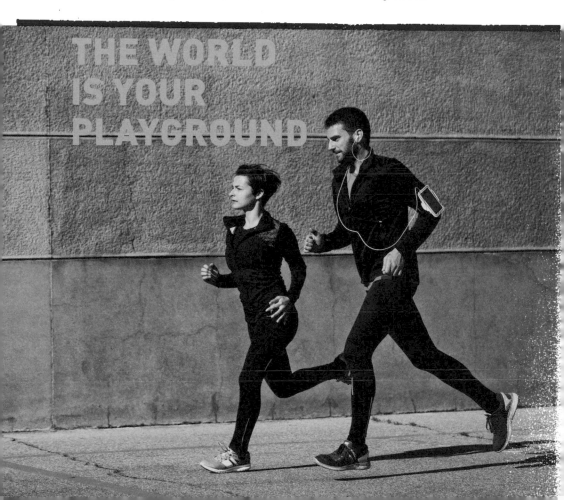

SO MANY MILES,

SO LITTLE TIME

It's tempting to put off quality mileage and training for Saturday and Sunday. The risk? You're cramming in too much distance, speed, or strength, or all three, in only two days. Overuse muscle injuries are not fun. If you're running long on Saturday and doing speed work on Sunday, your body will need a different amount of recovery than someone who sprinkles sessions in throughout the week.

- **Manage expectations.** Many race-training programs assume you're running three to five times a week. If you're following a training schedule like this but only running on Saturday and Sunday, you should reduce the total mileage so that you're increasing no more than 10 percent a week.

- **Monday–Friday aren't dead days.** Even if you don't have time to run, you still can find five to ten minutes to work on mobility, balance, or flexibility. Use a foam roller on your leg muscles while watching Hulu. Stand on one foot while washing dishes. Stand up and stretch during conference calls.

- **Warm up.** This is crucial to avoid injury. Don't be in a rush once you're finally getting to your run.

- **Diet matters.** The lower our activity levels, the lower our caloric burn, and the greater the need for proper fuel. Long work hours can lead to really poor eating habits. Plan ahead on Sunday. Make a big batch of food that you can portion for a few days for lunch or dinner.

- **Race accordingly.** If you haven't done the training, you shouldn't run the miles. If your goal is a marathon but you don't have the time for 20-milers right now, change your goal to a shorter race. Running your best 5K is damn satisfying and a much more reasonable time commitment.

DESTINATION RACES

THERE'S NO BETTER WAY TO SEE THE WORLD than with a pair of running shoes. From Berlin to Tokyo to Cambodia, I've let my legs take me around the world. I highly suggest destination races. You get to race, get a medal, and get to see a new place. Winning!

TIPS FOR TRAVELING TO RACES

1. If you're traveling to a new time zone, try to arrive either a week before or within two days of the race day to adjust to the time change. I find that either fully adjusting to a new time zone or letting adrenaline carry me is the best way to race. A weird three or four days in between leaves me sluggish.

2. Leave sightseeing for after the race. This seems counterintuitive, but walking after the race will leave you less sore and you won't be totally drained on race day if you leave that trek up the Eiffel Tower for afterward.

3. See if a local running store is hosting a shakeout run. Running tours are also common in a lot of cities.

4. Destination races are great opportunities to race for fun. Not every race should be a personal record. Some races are meant for high-fiving kids, taking selfies, and hamming it up.

5. Pack everything you need for race day in your carry-on. Under no circumstances should your race shoes be in your checked baggage! Remember, luggage gets lost and the last thing you want is to not have your running shoes on race day.

6. Have a game plan to get to the race and meet with any friends or family afterward. I spent two hours trying to find friends after the Amsterdam half marathon, with no phone, no plan, and no food. It wasn't cute. I got majorly lost in Paris on the way to the marathon because I took a wrong turn and had no map. Don't be me times two. Plan ahead and set up a meet-up location.

7. Check what your health insurance offers while you are abroad, in case something happens. If your insurance doesn't cover international travel, consider buying travel insurance with companies like Allianz or Travel Guard.

MY TIPS FOR STAYING FIT ON VACATION

1. Running shoes. Pack them. Lace up. Explore. Tourism on foot is awesome.

2. Hotel room workouts are the jam. Here's my favorite: high knees, squats, planks, crunches, push-ups, and dips. Do each exercise for 15 seconds, then 30, then 45, and then work your way back down to 15.

3. Do a pre-trip push. Get in extra miles or sessions before you head out. I'm obsessed with planning early morning sweat sessions the day I fly. Then I can read *US Weekly* while drinking red wine on a seventeen-hour flight and giving no f#%ks.

4. Adjust your expectations. You're on a vacation. Live a little. As long as the indulgence is temporary, you'll get back on track!

KEEP RUNNING INTERESTING

For many runners, you run the same routes around work or home to get the training done rather than travel to new routes, and while that makes for an easy run, it can also get boring. To stay motivated, here are some tips for keeping your run interesting.

1. ***Fartlek*** means "speed play" in Swedish and is a type of training run based on undefined intervals (like going back and forth between fast runs and slow runs). My favorite type of fartlek running is to alternate between jogging a block and sprinting a block. Before you know it, the run is over!

2. **Hit the trails.** If you're usually running in a town or city, find a trail through a park or nature preserve and explore. The softer surface will also give the bones and joints in your legs a break.

3. **Get some company.** The same route takes on new meaning with a friend, and knowing you have to meet someone will help motivate you.

4. **Commute to a new route.** It's worth the extra five to twenty minutes if your run will be enjoyable. Go to MapMyRun.com to see routes in your area that others have created.

TO-DO LIST:
BUILD MUSCLE.
BUILD WINGS.
BUILD DREAMS.

MAKE
YOURSELF
PROUD.

5. **Inject speed on your slower days.** The next time you find yourself feeling sluggish, bored, or struggling to go on a run, consider injecting a few speed bursts to reboot. Set your watch to 30 seconds and surge. Sometimes this shot of adrenaline is enough to ward off the blues.

6. **Expect a little boredom now and then.** We all experience it. The best way to get over a slump is to sign up for a race.

TRACK ATTACK

THE TRACK CAN BE INTIMIDATING, especially if you're not clocking elite-level times. Speed work is essential for any runner, whether you're competing with yourself or against others. Every time I hit the track, I have butterflies. The workouts are hard and the athletes around me look way more fit and way more intense. However, I never, ever regret it. You have to practice running fast in order to run faster, which means no matter how often you run, you should practice sprints and working on speed. Your body remembers what it feels like to soar and with that your form adjusts, oxygen capacity improves, and finish lines are conquered.

Not every speed session requires all-out sprints. Speed work can have varying goals. For example, a marathoner may attempt mile repeats, which is running one full mile around the track at race pace (four laps is equivalent to one mile), jogging for one lap, and then repeating any number of times. Alternatively, some sprints should be completed at your fastest pace and make you so breathless that you have no choice but to walk afterward.

TEN TRACK ETIQUETTE TIPS FOR NEWBIES

1. **Run counterclockwise.** Unless otherwise posted, run against the clock dial. Warm-ups and cooldowns are sometimes done clockwise in the outer lanes.

2. **Changing lanes.** The track is like a highway; fastest on the left and slowest on the right. The inside lanes (1 and 2) are intended for folks doing speed work. Recovery runs, warm-ups, and cooldowns should be done on the outer lanes. If a faster runner is coming up behind you, it's customary for them to yell "track" or "on your left" to give you a heads-up and let them pass. The outside lane is 40–50 meters longer than the inside lane. That's why some race starts are staggered.

3. **Space is at a premium.** Try to run no more than two abreast when running in a group. Be aware of stray elbows (keep them close to your body and at 90-degree angles, as mentioned on page 50). When you've done an interval, move out of the lane in case a runner is coming from behind.

4. **Leave the music at home.** It's important to be able to hear other runners, so if you're going to listen to music be sure to keep the volume low.

5. **Recovery is key.** Incorporate time at the end of a track workout for cooldown. Stopping abruptly is tough on the legs and the cardiovascular system.

6. **Fuel up.** Take in protein and carbs within 30 minutes of leaving the track. If you're commuting from the track, pack it with you.

7. **Rock your lightest kicks.** You don't need shoes with track spikes, but wearing shoes that are less than 10 ounces will give you a slight boost come race day. The lighter you are the faster you will move.

8. **Keeping track of your miles.** Many outdoor tracks are 400 meters. A mile is approximately 1,600 meters, or 4 laps. Half a mile is 800 meters, or 2 laps.

9. **Look "up track."** Just like crossing a street, look up the track for runners coming through while you run.

10. **Move drills and stretching to the infield.** Use the inner field or track perimeter to chill, stretch, and cooldown.

SUGGESTED SPEED WORKOUTS FOR EVERY RUNNER

Speed is relative and the elusive personal record (PR), or best time, is a carrot for most runners. The biggest mistake new or returning runners make is going out too fast. The second-biggest mistake is not going hard enough to get uncomfortable. The delicate dance between potential and pace is worth learning, and it takes trials, miles, and patience.

Striders: Increase your speed for 15–30 seconds toward the end of a run and repeat 3–10 times. This simulates sprinting to the finish at the end of the race.

Intervals: Timed intervals are the most accessible kind of speed work because everyone can assess a timing device. Intervals involve a period of high-intensity speed and recovery. The speed-to-recovery ratio makes the intervals tougher. Decrease your recovery to build oxygen capacity. If you're new to speed work, begin with 15-minute intervals and work up to as much as 60-minute intervals.

Many sport watches have an interval setting allowing you to time the intervals without much effort. Similarly, apps such as Seconds Pro have interval programs built in. The basic premise is to run fast for a period of time and then recover for a period of time.

Examples of interval workouts
- Mile repeats—one mile at race pace + ½-mile recovery
- 2-minute sprint + 1-minute recovery
- 1-minute sprint + 30-second recovery
- Sprint two blocks/between two lightposts/landmarks + jog two blocks/between two lightposts/landmarks

**THE
EXCUSES
THAT LIMIT
YOU ARE
ONLY THE
ONES YOU
ACCEPT.**

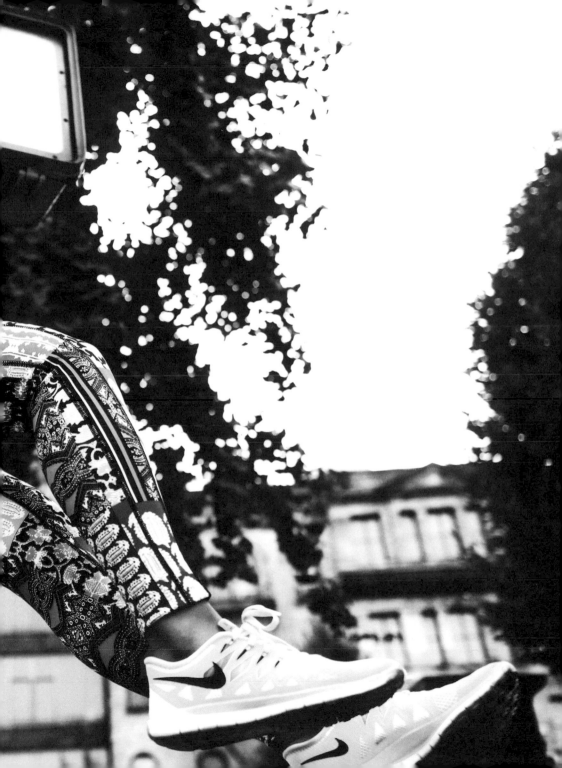

DON'T TREAD LIGHTLY

SPEED WORK on the treadmill isn't for everyone, but it's a great way to continue training in bad weather. The interval concept is the same on the treadmill: do an all-out run for a short time, recover for a few minutes at a slower pace, and then repeat. Remember, nothing actually replicates the elevation and environmental changes of running outside like . . . running outside. However, circumstances can make it difficult at times (namely weather), and it's always good to get in a run any way you can, especially if you're training for a race.

TREADMILL WORKOUTS

Intervals: Set the incline to 2.0. Sprint for 30 seconds. If you don't feel the need to walk at the end of 30 seconds, either increase the length of your sprint (45–60 seconds) or increase your speed. Sprint all out for 30 seconds and then walk or jog for 30. Repeat for 30 minutes.

Hills: Hill work is actually speed work. Lock in at a speed that feels like 50 percent exertion at 1.0 incline. The challenge for this session is to maintain that speed as you build up the hill. Every minute take the hill incline up by .5–1.0 until you reach a feeling of exertion at 80–90 percent. My favorite pattern is 5.0, 7.0, 10.0, 12.0, and back to 5.0. Think of yourself building up a ladder.

CHALLENGE: Pick one distance to attempt a personal record. Sign up for a race of that distance now, and then again in three months. Commit to once-weekly speed work with the goal of shaving off time. Remember, it can take a lot of work just to reduce your race pace by seconds. Keep your goals realistic and choose a shorter distance if you're new to racing.

HOW TO BEAT BOREDOM ON THE TREADMILL

I kind of hate the treadmill. I prefer to run outside any day, any time of the year, in any kind of weather. That said, there's utility and practicality in using a treadmill. Sometimes icy weather is just dangerous. While prepping for the Tokyo Marathon, I ran a 20-miler on a treadmill when there were inches of ice on the ground in New York City. When I was in Vietnam, the smog and traffic in Ho Chi Minh City made it impossible to run, so I used the hotel treadmill. I also regularly do Barry's Bootcamp—a combination cross-training and treadmill workout—for sprint work on the treadmill. I know the treadmill can be a buzzkill, so here are some helpful treadmill tips:

1. Use at least a 0.5 incline because otherwise you're essentially running downhill. I prefer locking in at 1.0 for a "flat" road run.

2. Go a little faster than your pace outside to stay on par with outdoor effort. For example, a ten-minute mile outside is more like 6.3 speed level on most treadmills, not 6.0 like the display calculates.

3. If you're bored, play with speed intervals or hill intervals (see page 69).

4. Compete with the person next to you.

5. If you're running but still feel like you're going nowhere, then work on your visualization. Sometimes our most boring, grueling workouts give us the juice necessary for tough parts of a race. Picture an upcoming racecourse or accomplishing a running goal.

6. Remember that you want to get your training in by any means necessary, so get it done!

7. Create a sick playlist.

TIME MANAGEMENT

LACK OF TIME IS THE BIGGEST EXCUSE people make for not sticking to a fitness plan. I get it. But at the end of the day, your life is your message and only you can create yourself. If you don't have enough time to work out, I challenge you to spend one day and account for every fifteen-minute interval. How much of that day was spent on Snapchat, Instagram, or watching television?

Countless times when I practiced law I had a set workout in my mind for after the workday. Suddenly the day would escape me and that particular workout I had planned was no longer possible. I came to realize that even a fifteen-minute jog between conference calls was better than sitting at my desk feeling sorry for myself while scrolling through Facebook. A little is always better than nothing.

If you only have a small window to run, use it. I believe short training sessions under 30 minutes should either be very hard or very easy. Set a timer on your watch, app, or phone. For a fifteen-minute all-out run, I recommend you sprint for 30 seconds, then jog for 30 seconds. Stop at lights to do squats and at every bench to do push-ups. If you don't have lights or benches, use a different visual marker, like every other house, tree, stop sign—you get the idea.

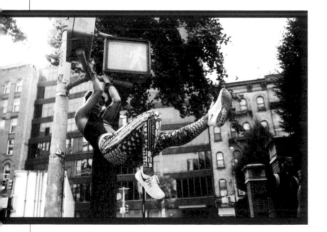

VISUALIZATION TIP

After your next solid run, I want you to write down how you felt below and then revisit it the next time you need motivation.

WHERE DID YOU RUN?
WHAT PART WAS THE HARDEST?
HOW DID YOU OVERCOME EXHAUSTION?
WHAT SONG WAS PLAYING?

Describe the run in detail. This will help remind you, when you'd rather sit on the couch or sleep in, how you feel after the hard work is done.

"YOU CAN'T FLIRT WITH THE TRACK, YOU MUST MARRY IT."

—BILL EASTON, SIX-TIME NCAA TITLE–WINNING TRACK COACH

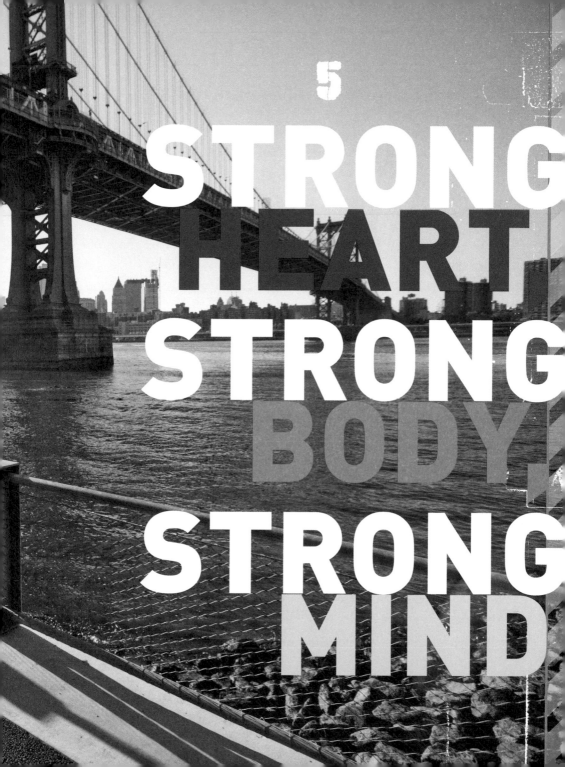

5

STRONG
HEART
STRONG
BODY,
STRONG
MIND

After I got a few marathons under my belt, I started to know my body. I knew the marathon hustle. I was also bored. Every running journey plateaus. At first, you might hit PR after PR as your body adjusts, but when the personal record magic starts to wane and it's just you at the thousandth mile, it can feel static. Plateaus are inevitable and part of the training process. They can even be a good thing when big life moments like weddings and babies and house moves are happening. Sometimes the name of the game is just maintenance. But if the momentum from the run starts to feel like inertia, here's how to stay in motion and revamp your running game.

STOP RUNNING

Hang up your shoes for a time and do some strength work. Trying new workouts is a win-win. If you love it, you have something else to add to your arsenal. If you hate it, you will appreciate your runs more. Start moving in different planes of motion, picking up and putting down some heavy shit, and stirring the pot. In the words of my homegirl and serious fitness queen Kira Stokes, "You have to shock it to rock it." So do something that doesn't involve running and remind your body what it means to be uncomfortable. If the thought of wearing spandex in a spin class makes you feel funny, then I say that's the first place you need to be. Good things never came from comfort zones unless it's a Netflix marathon of *Law & Order SVU*. The fitness industry is saturated and virtual, so even if you don't live in New York City, where a new studio opens every week around the corner from you, you can rock from home with resources like the DailyBurn, Peloton Cycle, and—this is huge—have you heard of this thing called YouTube?

IMPROVE YOUR BALANCE AND POSTURE

Lack of core strength and poor posture tend to go hand in hand. Unless you're tackling trail runs, you probably haven't done mobility and agility drills in a while (if ever). Even if you don't work at a desk, you probably sit and stare at some type of screen every day, which messes up your posture. Trust me.

Dabbling in Megaformer Pilates or yoga practice will not replace the runner's high, but it will strengthen your body with minimal pounding and increase your body awareness. The simple act of dropping your shoulders and activating your core can make or break your PR because your form is more efficient and less labored.

START A CHALLENGE

During the winter of 2014, I started a 5K-a-Day challenge with my friend Mishka Shubaly. I knew that if I challenged my Instagram followers to run a 5K every day of December I would be a complete jackass if I didn't do it, too. So I did. Your challenge doesn't have to be this extreme. Think of something that's feasible with your schedule, but that you actually don't really want to do, and then make it public. Get your homies in on the game or create a hashtag specific to the challenge so you can track the participation.

BUY SOME FIERCE GEAR

Sometimes it's just about buying new gear. I literally don't care how vain this sounds because trust me, it works. And it's not just about the ladies.

TRACK METRICS

Get some gadgets to make movement a game. If you're used to logging distance and speed, play with logging different metrics like heart rate, cadence, and elevation training. There's something for every price point, from Jawbone to Fitbit to Garmin.

RUN FOR CHARITY

Nothing will give your run more purpose than when it's about someone or something you care about. Racing for MS research changed my life, and that's not hyperbole. It's important that the cause is something meaningful because when you're asking people for money you want to be able to tell an authentic story as to why you're doing it. You don't personally need to know someone that the nonprofit is helping but it helps to have an emotional connection to the cause you're racing for.

FORM A RAGNAR RELAY TEAM (www.ragnarrelay.com)

Ragnar Relay is a 200-mile relay with a team of twelve people. They are all over the United States and provide insane amounts of fun with minimal training. Each runner covers three legs, over 24 hours, totaling 10–20 miles. These runs are not about your PR, but your team's mission, namely, dressing up and having fun. You're delirious from the 24-hour race and it's worth it.

SIGN UP FOR AN ULTRAMARATHON

I'm a firm believer that a race on the horizon is always a good idea. If you're in a slump then maybe you forget the PR-chasing and just focus on willing your body to complete an epic distance. Technically, an "ultramarathon" is any race longer than 26.2 miles. Common ultra distances are 50K (approximately 31 miles), 50 miles, 100 miles, and stage races, which are a combination of 50+ miles over 5–7 days totally 150+ miles. The running community is special and the ultra community is the icing on the cake. Some of the kindest and most awe-inspiring runners I've met are ultra endurance athletes (no shade to the sprinters). So, sign up for an ultra if you want to rock the shit out of your running, your core, your soul, and set your life on fire (big sell?). Even if you're a seasoned ultra runner, you can always find an awesome new course.

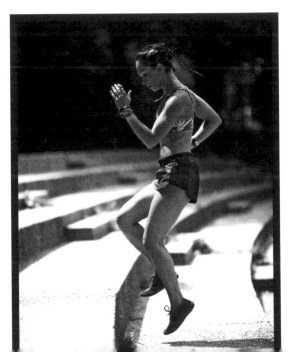

CHALLENGE: Change up your workout routine and schedule a new class every week for a month, ranging from boot camps to spin to rowing to a high-intensity interval training (HIIT) class.

TRANSITIONING TO ULTRAMARATHON RUNNING FROM 26.2

SURPRISINGLY, running a 50K or 50-miler isn't drastically different than training for a marathon. If you can complete a marathon then you can complete an ultra. Some sage advice is that you should be running for X amount of years or miles before attempting an ultra—but I call bullshit. If you're willing to put in the time to train and learn how to fuel properly, then you can do it. The transition from marathon to ultramarathon also assumes you're just trying to finish the ultra, and not break a record. However, those who win ultramarathons still do speed work and all the other crazy things that are required of champions.

- The 10 Percent rule still applies to ultra training. Jumping more than 10 percent in cumulative distance a week risks injury, so plan a race far enough out so that you hit 60+ miles a week before the race. While weekly mileage is really dependent on the runner, plan on adding 20 miles of running a week at a minimum, which then means you need to leave yourself at least three months of training time in addition to a base training period where you are building weekly mileage. You can and should piggyback on marathon training for ultras in the same season if you're not injured.

- The linchpin of ultra training is back-to-back long runs, meaning a typical marathon training run (26.2 miles) on a Saturday and then either a slightly shorter or slightly longer distance on a Sunday. This teaches your body to run on tired legs without having to do the entire ultra distance before race day. Marathon training rarely requires running the actual distance before race day and ultras are no different, but long runs done within twelve hours of each other simulate running on tired legs. For a 50-mile race, you should peak at 30 miles a month before the race.

- Running and walking is totally kosher in ultras, even by extremely fit people. Running a race without walking is an amazing goal for shorter distances, but that's not realistic for most ultra athletes. The key for ultras is logging time on your feet. Many training runs prior to an ultramarathon are about hours, not miles.

- You must learn to eat on the run. And, no, you will not be able to rely on energy gels for an entire 50-mile race. Training for an ultra involves long runs as much as it involves eating actual, real food. Variety is key because what works at 6 a.m. might not stay down or taste good when you're running ten hours later. Common foods at ultramarathons are energy bars, pretzels, chips, boiled potatoes, chicken soup, every variety of sandwich cookies, crackers, bananas, and oranges.

- Most ultras are on trails or rough terrain, so you might need to invest in gear such as trail shoes with a rock plate (part of a shoe sole that protects from the impact of landing on rocks) and/or a headlamp.

- Hill work is crucial because many ultras are on trails that usually involve serious mountain elevation. Check the technical requirements of a course before signing up. I love the North Face Endurance Challenge series because the courses are well marked and are often held on beautiful mountains. Ultramarathon pros even walk up steep inclines to get their legs used to tackling different elevations and you should, too.

- Under no circumstances should your significant other, friends, and/or family pace you at your first ultra unless they know what they are getting into. Running an ultra will likely take you to some intense emotional places and you might take your exhaustion out on them.

- Your pace will be slower than normal, but that's to be expected. Crossing the finish of an ultra is some boss shit, and trust me when I say you're not going to care if it's possibly minutes slower per mile than your marathon pace. This doesn't mean forgo speed work during training. Speed work does have a place in ultra training, but it should take a big backseat to distance if you have to choose between the two.

- Recovery is going to be key. The days of "not stretching" on a rest day are gone. You must do it to keep your muscles limber.

TRAINING PLANS

HERE ARE MY TRAINING PLANS to help you prepare for a 5K, 10K, a half marathon, marathon, and a 50-mile race. Generally, these programs involve a two-week build followed by one-week recovery involving a decrease in mileage. Virtually every training plan you'll find follows this to varying degrees. If it doesn't feel right, then don't do it! Blindly following any training plan is stupid. Yes, you will be uncomfortable and probably sore. No, you shouldn't run with the flu or a bone sticking out of your leg.

Training plans are not static. If your best day to rest is different than prescribed on the following pages, then change your training to make it work. The training you make time for is infinitely better than the training that falls off because the plan doesn't fit with your schedule. Remember, it's okay to take additional rest days, but take the rest you need, not the rest you want. There's a difference.

NEED TO KNOW

1. Before every run, take five minutes to jog or briskly walk to warm up your legs and to get the endorphins flowing.

2. **Your training key**
   ST = Striders, a type of speed work where you increase your stride length at the end of the run. Striders help to improve your form. In the final quarter or half mile (depending on whether it's marked ¼ or ½), alternate picking up the pace for 20–30 second bursts (or a few blocks) and then back down to your comfortable pace.
   RP = your ideal race pace.
   XT = cross-training such as cycling or weight lifting.
   Tempo = A comfortably hard pace (6 out of 10 effort). You should feel like you're pushing your limit, but not all out sprinting.

3. This is what it means to run easy: when you can pass the talk test. Can you sing a verse of your favorite song or talk to a friend during the run? Good. Maintain that conversational pace throughout the entire run. You don't want to burn out early.

4. Start with a fixed-timed run to build a base. Don't worry about mileage or your pace until specified in each plan.

FROM THE COUCH TO YOUR FIRST 5K IN 7 WEEKS

THE NUMBER-ONE MISTAKE NEW RUNNERS MAKE? Going out too fast, getting frustrated, and stopping. Resist the urge to sprint out of the gate. Your pacing will come. Just focus on getting out there and being consistent. Avoid skipping ahead or compounding workouts if you miss a day. Above all, *listen* to your body and remember you are capable of extraordinary things. Enjoy the journey!

M	T	W	Th	F	S	Su
WEEK 1: This week gives you the option to run or walk for a specified period of time. The only day you should track your distance is Sunday. The other days are for time only.						
Walk/run for 20 minutes	Walk for 20 minutes	Rest	Walk/run for 25 minutes	Walk/run for 25 minutes	Rest	Walk/run for 3 miles (no matter how long it takes)
WEEK 2: Just like week 1, week 2 gives you the option to run or walk for a specified period of time. Again, the only day you should track your distance is Sunday. The others days are for time only.						
Walk/run for 30 minutes	Walk for 30 minutes	Walk/run for 25 minutes	Rest	Walk/run for 30 minutes	Rest	Run for 3.5 miles
WEEK 3: Same as the last two weeks. Run or walk for a specified period of time. The only day you should track your distance is Sunday.						
Walk/run for 30 minutes	Walk for 40 minutes	Rest	Walk/run for 30 minutes	Walk/run for 30 minutes	Walk/run for 20 minutes	Run for 2.5 miles
WEEK 4: You are now one month into training and it's time to start to err on the side of jogging over walking. This is also a lower-mileage week so take advantage of the shorter workouts. Push your limits.						
Run for 25 minutes	Jog for 30 minutes	Rest	Run for 30 minutes	Run for 20 minutes	Rest	Run for 3 miles

KEEP IT GOING →

M	T	W	Th	F	S	Su
WEEK 5: Time to pick up the pace.						
Run for 35 minutes	Jog for 45 minutes	Rest	Run for 30 minutes	Run for 35 minutes	Run for 25 minutes	Run for 4 miles
WEEK 6: Keep it up!						
Run for 35 minutes	Jog for 40 minutes	Run for 30 minutes	Run for 30 minutes	Rest	Run for 25 minutes	Run for 4.5 miles
WEEK 7: Race week! Trust your training. If you missed a session, now is not the time to make it up.						
Run for 30 minutes	Walk for 30 minutes	Rest	Run for 30 minutes	Walk for 30 minutes	Rest	**5K RACE**

PROCEED AS IF SUCCESS IS THE ONLY OPTION.

TRAINING FOR A 10K IN 12 WEEKS

	M	T	W	Th	F	S	Su
WEEK 1							
	XT	20-minute easy run	30-minute easy run	Rest	Rest or XT	35-minute easy run	35-minute easy run
WEEK 2							
	XT	25-minute easy run	30-minute easy run	Rest	Rest or XT	40-minute easy run	Rest
WEEK 3							
	XT	30-minute easy run	30-minute easy run	Rest	Rest or XT	35-minute easy run	Rest
WEEK 4: You are now one month into training. Time to transition from runs based on minutes to runs based on miles.							
	XT	3 miles easy run	4–5 miles easy run	Rest	XT	4 miles easy run	Rest
WEEK 5							
	XT	3.5 miles easy run	4 miles easy run	Rest	2.5 miles easy run	6 miles easy run	3 miles easy run
WEEK 6							
	XT	2 miles easy run	4–5 miles, ST ¼, pick up the pace for a quarter-mile strider* at the end of the run.	Rest	3 miles easy run	5 miles, ST ¼	3 miles easy run

Reminder, the strider should be faster than your average running pace, but not an all-out sprint.

KEEP IT GOING →

	M	T	W	Th	F	S	Su
WEEK 7							
	XT	3 miles easy run	4–5 mile run, ST ¼	Rest	3 miles easy run	7 mile run, ST ¼	3 miles easy run
WEEK 8: By week 8, your Friday runs should be ran at your RP (race pace). See the training key on page 83 as a reference.							
	XT	2 miles easy run	5 miles, ST ¼	Rest	3 miles RP	5 miles, ST ½	5 miles easy run
WEEK 9							
	XT	3 miles easy run	4–5 miles, ST ¼	Rest	2 miles RP	8 miles, ST ¼	4 miles easy run
WEEK 10							
	XT	3.5 miles easy run	4–5 miles, ST ¼	Rest	2 miles RP	7 miles, ST ¼	4–5 miles easy run
WEEK 11							
	XT	3 miles easy run	3–4 miles, ST ¼	Rest	2 miles RP	4 miles, ST ½	3–5 miles easy run
WEEK 12							
	XT	2 miles easy run	3–4 miles easy run	2 miles RP	Rest or 2 miles easy run	**RACE DAY**	Rest

TRAINING FOR A HALF MARATHON (13.1 MILES)

A HALF MARATHON ISN'T JUST ABOUT THE DISTANCE. It's about crossing the finish line stronger than when you started the journey. Before you start this program, you should be able to comfortably run at an easy pace for 45 minutes or 4 miles. Check out the 10K plan if you'd like a primer. Listen to your body and shatter limitations. If you tell your mind, your body will follow. Welcome to the road to 13.1!

M	T	W	Th	F	S	Su
WEEK 1						
3–4 miles easy run	XT	4 miles easy run	3 miles easy run	Rest/Yoga	6 miles run	Rest
WEEK 2						
4 miles easy run	XT	4 miles easy run	3 miles easy run	Rest/Yoga	6 miles run	Rest
WEEK 3						
3 miles easy run	XT	4 miles easy run	4 miles easy run	Rest/Yoga	7 miles run	Rest
WEEK 4						
5 miles easy run	XT	3 miles easy run	4 miles easy run	Rest/Yoga	5 miles run	Rest
WEEK 5: By week 5, incorporate tempo runs into your training. See the training key on page 83 as a reference.						
4 miles easy run	XT	5 miles easy run	4 miles tempo	Rest/Yoga	8 miles run	Rest

KEEP IT GOING →

	M	T	W	Th	F	S	Su
WEEK 6							
	4 miles easy run	XT	5 miles, tempo	4 miles, tempo	Rest/Yoga	9–10 miles run	Rest
WEEK 7							
	5 miles easy run	XT	4 miles, tempo	5 miles easy run	Rest/Yoga	11 miles run	Rest
WEEK 8							
	5 miles easy run	XT	5 miles, tempo	4 miles easy run	Rest/Yoga	12 miles run	Rest
WEEK 9							
	5 miles easy run	XT	4 miles, tempo	5 miles easy run	Rest/Yoga	9 miles run	Rest
WEEK 10							
	5 miles RP	XT	4 miles, tempo	4 miles easy run	Rest/Yoga	10 miles run	Rest
WEEK 11							
	5 miles RP	XT	4 miles, tempo	5 miles easy run	Rest/Yoga	8 miles run	Rest
WEEK 12							
	4 miles easy run	4 miles RP	3 miles easy run	4 miles easy run	Rest	**RACE DAY!**	Rest

TRAINING FOR A MARATHON (26.2 MILES)

BY THE TIME YOU VENTURE TO TRAINING FOR A MARATHON, you should be able to run for 45 minutes without stopping. This plan assumes that even if you haven't raced a shorter distance, you have a base number of weekly miles and conditioning. If you're not running more than 15–20 miles a week, check out the 10K plan and build your base first.

WHAT SHOULD THE RUNS FEEL LIKE?

Easy: 70–80% of your weekly marathon training mileage should be done at an easy conversational pace.

Intervals: Generally done at your 5K pace unless otherwise specified.

Fartlek: a type of training run based on undefined intervals (i.e., sprinting mixed with jogging).

Yasso 800s: Speed work that entails repeated effort for 800 meters followed by recovery.

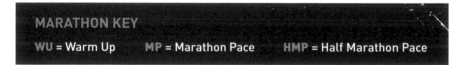

MARATHON KEY

WU = Warm Up   **MP** = Marathon Pace   **HMP** = Half Marathon Pace

ABS AND STRENGTH

Pick three exercises from each and do three sets of each for 8–10 repetitions.

Legs: single leg squats; dead lift with weights; squats with weights; lunges with weights; hamstring curls; lying hip twist; split squats; side lunges; or squat jumps.

Core: plank (three times for one minute each); side plank (thirty seconds on each side four times); bicycle crunches; toe touches; Russian twists with weights; medicine ball wood chop; tabata; bridge; oblique crunch.

Upper Body: pushups; chin-ups; shoulder presses; bench press; pushups on a BOSU ball; bicep curls; or chest fly.

M	T	W	Th	F	S	Su
WEEK 1						
4 miles easy run followed by abs and strength	2-mile WU; 5 x hill repeat, find an incline and repeat the climb, up and down, 5 times or a total of one mile; 2-mile cooldown	5 miles easy run followed by abs and strength	7 miles tempo - 2-miles WU run, 3 miles at 5K pace, and 2-mile cooldown	XT, focus on abs and strength	9 miles MP run	Rest
WEEK 2						
4 miles easy run; finish with ST (20–40 second speed bursts) x 4	5 x hill repeats; find an incline and repeat the climb, up and down, 5 times or a total of one mile.	6 miles easy run followed by abs and strength	Interval - 3 one-mile repeats at MP	Rest	10 miles MP run; finish with ST (20–40 second speed bursts) x 4	Rest
WEEK 3						
5 miles easy run followed by abs and strength	Fartlek - 8 miles; 1-mile WU; 6-miles alternating 5K pace for 5 minutes and MP for 5 minutes; 1-mile cooldown	7 miles easy run followed by abs and strength	4 miles easy run	Rest	11 miles MP run	Rest

KEEP IT GOING →

M	T	W	Th	F	S	Su
WEEK 4						
8 miles easy run finish with ST (20–40 second speed bursts) x 4 followed by abs and strength	Track - 8 x 1200 meters alternating between 800M at MP and 400M at your goal marathon pace within each repeat. Take no recovery between the components of the repeat.	6 miles easy run; finish with ST (20–40 second speed bursts) x 4	5 miles easy run	Rest	13 miles easy run followed by abs and strength	Rest
WEEK 5						
8 miles easy run followed by abs and strength	Track - 2-mile WU; 20–24 x 200M with 200M jog at 5K to 10K pace; 2-mile cooldown	10 miles easy run; finish with ST (20–40 second speed bursts) x 4	XT	8 miles easy run followed by abs and strength	15 miles MP run	Rest
WEEK 6						
9 miles easy run followed by abs and strength	Track - YASSO 800s: 10 x 800M with 3 minute recovery; 2-mile WU and 2-mile cooldown	8 miles easy run followed by abs and strength	Tempo - 2-mile WU; 20 minutes comfortably hard (faster than 10K pace); 2-miles cooldown	4 miles easy run; finish with ST (20–40 second speed bursts) x 4	11 miles MP run	Rest

KEEP IT GOING →

	M	T	W	Th	F	S	Su
WEEK 7							
	5 miles easy run followed by abs and strength	Tempo - 2-mile WU; 4 miles faster than 10K pace; 2-mile cooldown	9 miles easy run followed by abs and strength	Intervals - 2-mile WU; 8 x 200M starting at 5K pace to sprint with 200M recovery; 2-mile cooldown	7 miles easy run	12 miles MP run; finish with ST (20–40 second speed bursts) x 4	Rest
WEEK 8							
	8 miles easy run; finish with ST (20–40 second speed bursts) x 4	Intervals - 2 miles WU run; 4 x one-mile starting at 10K pace, ending at 5K with three minute rests between sets. 2-mile cooldown.	10 miles easy run followed by abs and strength	8 miles easy run; finish with ST (20–40 second speed bursts) x 4	4 miles easy run	15 miles MP run	Abs and strength
WEEK 9							
	8 miles easy run	Intervals - YASSO 800s: 10 x 800M with 3 minute recovery; 2-mile WU and cooldown	10 miles easy run followed by abs and strength	6 miles Tempo run - 2-mile WU; 5 x 800M at HMP; 5 x 800M at 10K pace; 2-mile cooldown	Abs and strength	16 miles MP run	Rest

KEEP IT GOING $\longrightarrow$

M	T	W	Th	F	S	Su
WEEK 10						
6 miles easy run followed by abs and strength	Intervals - 2-mile WU; 3 x 1600M at 10K pace; 3 x 400M at 5K pace; rest two minutes between reps and three minutes between sets. 2-mile cooldown	9 miles easy run followed by abs and strength	5 miles Tempo run - 2-mile WU; 3 miles alternating 800M at HMP and 800M at 10K pace	Rest	18 miles MP run	Rest
WEEK 11						
5 miles easy run; finish with ST (20–40 second speed bursts) x 4	10 miles easy run followed by abs and strength	Tempo - 2-mile WU; 4 miles at HMP; 2-mile cooldown	5 miles easy run followed by abs and strength	XT	Rest	20 miles easy run
WEEK 12						
Rest	Intervals - 8–10 x 400M with 200M jog at HMP, 10K, 5K, and 3K race pace	6 miles easy run, abs and strength	8 miles easy run; Tempo: WU for 2; 4 miles faster than 10K pace; 2-mile cooldown	4 miles easy run followed by abs and strength	Rest	13 miles run

KEEP IT GOING ⟶

DREAM WHILE YOU'RE AWAKE.

	M	T	W	Th	F	S	Su
WEEK 13							
	3 miles easy run	Intervals – 4 x one-mile repeats with 400M recovery. Start at HMP and finish at 10K pace.	4 miles easy run	7 miles easy run followed by abs and strength	Rest	3 miles MP run	6 miles easy run
WEEK 14							
	4 miles easy run	Rest	Rest	5 miles easy run	Rest	2 miles easy run	**RACE DAY**

TRAINING FOR 50 MILES IN 20 WEEKS

WHEN VENTURING INTO ULTRAMARATHON TERRITORY you have to remember one thing: sometimes to go fast you have to go slow. A solid initial goal for any new distance should be to finish rocking your invisible crown with your head held high and injury-free. The below plan incorporates two recovery days on Mondays and Fridays. If you need to run in the morning and night to get the mileage in that's okay, but don't sacrifice the long run! These are essential, even more so than in marathon training. If you need to take some long runs in hours not miles, that's okay, too. Many ultra training plans are based on time rather than distance as long as you are covering at least a marathon distance during training. In fact, it's a good idea to run a marathon during training but not for time! Exercise the discipline of holding back knowing the larger finish is on the horizon. Happy running, Baby. Welcome to less than .5% of the world who have done this.

	M	T	W	Th	F	S	Su
WEEK 1							
	Rest	Run 3 miles	Run 6 miles	Run 3 miles	Rest	Run 15 miles	Run 6 miles
WEEK 2							
	Rest	3 miles	6 miles	3 miles	Rest	18 miles	6 miles
WEEK 3: This is a down week so rest and repair accordingly, even if that means skipping a 3-mile run.							
	Rest	3 miles	5 miles	3 miles	Rest	8 miles	5 miles
WEEK 4							
	Rest	3 miles	7 miles	3 miles	Rest	20 miles	8 miles
WEEK 5: Incorporate striders at the end of your midweek short runs. Next week we decrease mileage again, so go hard this week.							
	Rest	4 miles	7 miles	3 miles	Rest	20 miles	10 miles

KEEP IT GOING →

	M	T	W	Th	F	S	Su
WEEK 6							
	Rest	4 miles	5 miles	4 miles	Rest	10 miles	8 miles
WEEK 7							
	Rest	4 miles	6 miles	6 miles	Rest	22 miles	10 miles
WEEK 8							
	Rest	4 miles	10 miles	6 miles	Rest	22 miles	12 miles
WEEK 9							
	Rest	4 miles	5 miles	6 miles	Rest	12 miles	10 miles
WEEK 10: You're reaching the point in training where long runs reach 24+ miles. Find a marathon to run during the next month. Adjust the training schedule accordingly to incorporate that race day. For example, if the race is next week then run 26 miles instead of 24, and run the 24-mile distance the weekend after. It's also okay to do these longer runs in hours instead of distance as long as you're running for a minimum of 3.5+ hours a run.							
	Rest	4 miles	9 miles	7 miles	Rest	24 miles	10 miles
WEEK 11							
	Rest	4 miles	8 miles	7 miles	Rest	24 miles	10 miles
WEEK 12							
	Rest	5 miles	6 miles	6 miles	Rest	10 miles	10 miles
WEEK 13							
	Rest	4 miles	9 miles	6 miles	Rest	Marathon or 5-hour run	10 miles

KEEP IT GOING ⟶

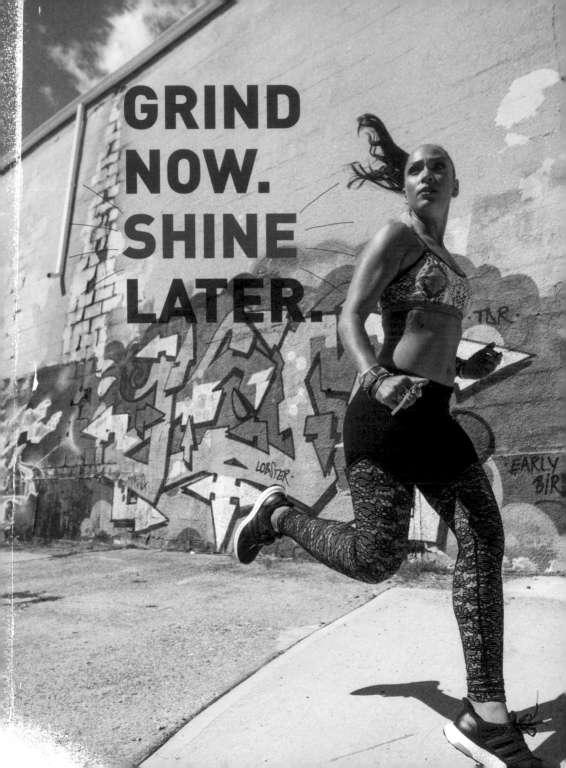

	M	T	W	Th	F	S	Su
WEEK 14							
	Rest	4 miles	10 miles	7 miles	Rest	Marathon or 5-hour run	10 miles
WEEK 15							
	Rest	4 miles	8 miles	6 miles	Rest	12 miles	8 miles
WEEK 16: Your training peaks this week and next. Do not try to make up runs you haven't done. Take an honest assessment of your training.							
	Rest	4 miles	14 miles	8 miles	Rest	28 miles	12 miles
WEEK 17: Another peak training week. Again, do not try to make up runs you've missed. Take an honest assessment of your training.							
	Rest	4 miles	14 miles	8 miles	Rest	28 miles	12 miles
WEEK 18: Taper starts now. This is not the time to go hard with speed or make up long runs. It's better to be slightly undertrained than overtrained and potentially injured.							
	Rest	4 miles	8 miles	7 miles	Rest	10 miles	10 miles
WEEK 19							
	Rest	5 miles	Rest	7 miles	Rest	12 miles	Rest
WEEK 20: It's race week! Leave your metrics at home. Run on feeling. Err on the side of skipping a run if you need the rest but do not be a couch potato. It's important to keep the blood volume up!							
	Run for an hour. Distance doesn't matter.	Run for 45 minutes. Distance doesn't matter.	Run for 30 minutes. Distance doesn't matter.	Rest	Rest (2-mile shakeout if you're going crazy).	**50 MILES, BABY**	MAJOR REST

LACE UP.

THOSE AREN'T SNEAKERS, THEY'RE INSTRUMENTS IN YOUR LIBERATION.

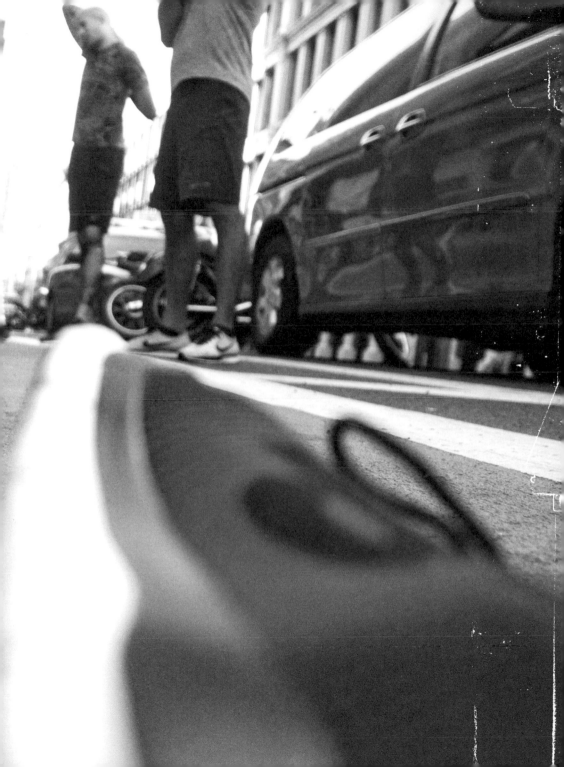

IT'S OKAY TO WANT IT ALL IF YOU'RE WILLING TO WORK FOR IT.

HERE ARE MY TIPS FOR A STRONG RACE DAY

1. **Nothing new on race day.** Try out new clothes, shoes, pacing, and nutrition on your training runs, but not on race day.

2. **Mind over miles.** Eighty percent of the battle to the finish is mental.

3. **Trust the training.** It works. Really.

4. **Don't skip long runs.** Missing a short run here and there to recover or because you got too drunk the night before is okay. But long runs are essential to getting your body used to performing when it's tired.

5. **Listen to your body.** I'm all about pushing your limits, but listen to your body so you can tell when you need to pull back. There's impending injury and then there's being a wuss.

6. **Leave the iPod at home.** Music can be a great motivation, but do some runs without music to learn how to listen to your breathing and learn your natural cadence.

7. **Put your name on your shirt.** Race day crowds can make a race. Let them sing your praises.

8. **Get the right shoes.** Kicks that worked for a 5K might not work for marathon training. Get a gait analysis at your local running store to make sure you're in the right shoes for each distance.

9. **Chafing sucks.** Use some type of lube (like Body Glide) over any parts of your body that might chafe. This means inner thighs, arms, feet, and, for guys, nipples.

10. **Roll out.** Keep your muscles limber. I swear by yoga and a foam roller. Ten minutes a day can keep injury away.

BUCKET LIST RACES

5K/10K
- [ ] **Red Hook Criterium 5K** (Brooklyn)
- [ ] **Hot Chocolate 5K** (Chicago)
- [ ] Any **turkey trot** around Thanksgiving. There's nothing like breaking a sweat before getting ready to feast with family.
- [ ] **Run for Your Lives**—an obstacle course where you're chased by zombies (locations in United States, Europe, Asia, and Australia).
- [ ] **Empire State Building** (New York City)—not a 5K, but a dope climb of 1,576 stairs up an iconic building.
- [ ] **World's Best 10K** (San Juan, Puerto Rico)
- [ ] **Cooper River Bridge Run 10K** (South Carolina)
- [ ] **Beach to Beacon 10K** (Cape Elizabeth, Maine)
- [ ] **Bay to Breakers** (San Francisco)

Half Marathon (13.1 miles)
- [ ] **Star Wars Half Marathon Disneyland** (Anaheim, California)
- [ ] **Brooklyn Half Marathon** (Brooklyn)
- [ ] **Staten Island Half Marathon** (Staten Island)—seriously, this race is fun! The crowd support is awesome, the ferry ride is amazing, and people are psyched for the New York City Marathon just weeks away. Also, it's the home of Wu-Tang Clan. So, yeah.
- [ ] **Napa to Sonoma Wine Country Half Marathon** (Sonoma, California)
- [ ] **ZOOMA Cape Cod Half Marathon** (North Falmouth, Massachusetts)
- [ ] **Superhero Half Marathon** (Morris, New Jersey)

Marathon (26.2 miles)
- [ ] **New York City Marathon**—my favorite race on the planet. I've never received more love from a racecourse. New York is my boyfriend, after all.
- [ ] **Berlin Marathon**
- [ ] **Tokyo Marathon**
- [ ] **Big Sur International Marathon** (Big Sur, California)
- [ ] **Great Wall Marathon** (east of Beijing, China)
- [ ] **Australian Outback Marathon** (Ayers Rock, Australia)
- [ ] **Serengeti Marathon** (Tanzania)
- [ ] **Boston Marathon**

Ultramarathon (anything more than 26.2 miles)
- [ ] every **North Face Endurance Challenge** race
- [ ] **Burning Man Ultramarathon** (Black Rock City, Nevada), 50 miles
- [ ] **Rocky 50K Fat Ass Run** (Philadelphia), 50 miles
- [ ] **Comrades Marathon** (KwaZulu-Natal Province of South Africa), 56 miles
- [ ] **Marathon des Sables** (Sahara Desert in southern Morocco), 156 miles
- [ ] **EPIC5 Challenge** (Hawaii)
- [ ] **Badwater Ultramarathon** (Badwater Basin in California), 135 miles
- [ ] **Leadville Trail 100 Run** (Leadville, Colorado), 100 miles

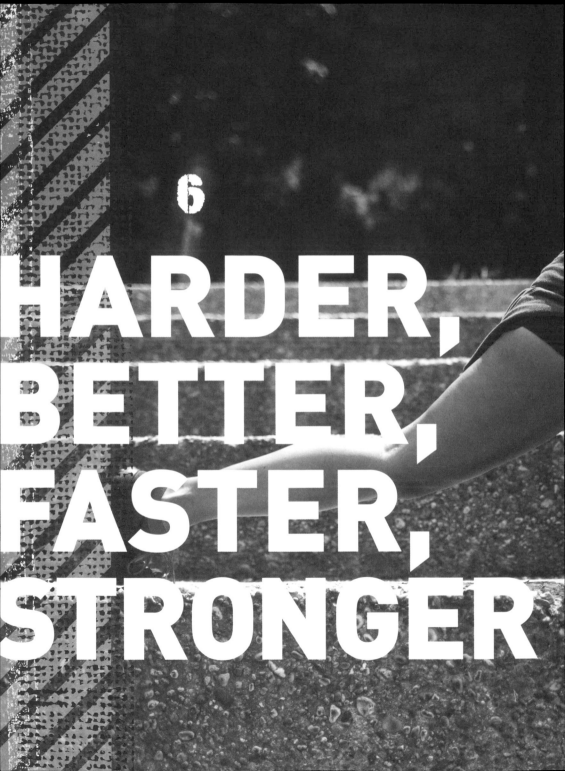

6

HARDER, BETTER, FASTER, STRONGER

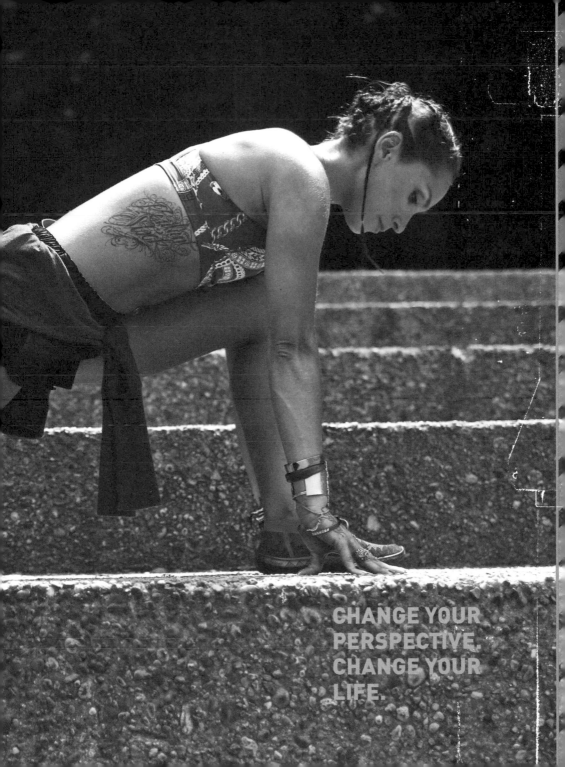

CHANGE YOUR
PERSPECTIVE.
CHANGE YOUR
LIFE.

WHEN IN DOUBT, PLANK IT OUT

I KNOW TOO MANY RUNNERS who neglect strength work. Yes, you have to run to be able to run, but the more you can push and pull your own body weight the more efficient you will be on the road and racecourse. The number-one strength move I swear by targets the core. The muscles in your abdominals, lower back, and glutes provide the stability and power that runners need. These postural muscles are even more important toward the end of a race, when fatigue sets in and form suffers.

Quality core work doesn't require equipment or even a lot of time. Consistency is key.

Incorporate planks 3–4 times a week for 5–15 minutes.

1. **The Basic Plank:** Spend time feeling comfortable in a basic plank before getting fancy with it. Start by getting into a push-up position. Bend your elbows and rest your weight on your forearms, not your hands. Squeeze your gluts to stabilize your body. Your body should form a straight line from shoulders to ankles. There are no peaks or valley, meaning your butt shouldn't reach for the sky and your lower back shouldn't dip toward the ground. Be careful not to lock out your knees. If you feel discomfort in your lower back or shoulders, you can start this move with your knees on the ground. You should feel energy coming through your legs and out your heels. Engage your core by activating your belly. This doesn't mean suck in your belly and hold your breathe! Think about how you would react if someone were about to punch you in the gut. For a lighter example, think about how your stomach reacts to a cough or a laugh. You prepare by bracing your midsection and creating a solid ring of muscles around your belly. Hold the position for 30 seconds. Relax. Repeat. Gradually increase the time of your plank as you get stronger.

2. **Side Plank:** This variation of the plank better engages your obliques (the side muscles of the abdomen). Once in the plank position, turn your body to one side with your elbow directly below your shoulder on the ground, stack your legs on top of one another, and raise your hips to the sky. If you need more support, you can modify by bending one knee on the ground. An advanced version of this move is to raise the opposing arm or leg in the air.

There are tons of ways to work your core. I don't believe in reinventing the wheel. Planks work. Now you just have to do them. Set a timer. Put on some jams. Go!

HOW TO BECOME A MORNING RUNNER

SUNRISE RUNS are some of the most glorious runs possible. They are also a complete bitch for some of us to get up for. I was never a morning runner until I started coaching 6 a.m. spin classes. I don't drink coffee, never have, so I don't use caffeine to get me out of bed. If sheer will and determination don't do it for you, here are some tips for becoming a morning runner. When you fall off, and you will, try again. Afterward, you'll feel great knowing you did more than most people do all day, and forming the habit will make it easier. Keep going!

- Lay out your gear the night before or sleep in it. Seriously. Destroy any impediment or excuse. The less you have to do the faster you will lace up and get out the door.

- Meet a friend. Knowing someone is waiting for you will get your ass out of bed.

- Disable snooze on your alarm. Snooze is the devil. While you're at it, change the subject of your alarm header on your smartphone to say something that motivates you. "Get after it" works for me.

- Place your alarm clock out of arm's reach. If you have to physically get out of bed to turn the alarm off then you're less likely to go back to sleep.

- Set one alarm that gets you up and another that gets you out the door. Leave yourself enough time to brush your teeth, hydrate, eat a little something, and bounce. No dawdling.

- If you drink coffee, set your coffeemaker to brew before your alarm goes off. The smell might entice you to get up!

- If you have a partner, get him or her on board to kick your ass out of bed.

- When the alarm goes off, sit up. If you can sit up, you can get up. Let this be your mantra for early morning runs!

- Read something running related before bed. If running is the last conscious thought you have before bed, sometimes it's enough inspiration to carry over to dawn.

- Warm up. Turn on some jams and dance in your kitchen. This will wake up your mind and your muscles. Beyoncé is a personal favorite of mine.

STAYING SAFE AT NIGHT

IF YOU KNOW you'll never give up your snooze button and you're the type who would pay money to sleep in for five more minutes, then you probably prefer to run at night. If that's the case, here are some tips for staying safe.

• Tell someone you're going for a run even if you live alone. Apps like Glympse or RunSafe allow you to share your location for up to four hours.

• No headphones, or else keep the music on low. Music can distract you from your surroundings and can make you an easy target.

• Run a route you know so there's zero risk of getting lost.

• Bring a phone.

• Run with someone.

• Wear bright clothing or reflective gear. If you're in a super-remote area run with a headlamp.

• Run against traffic so you can see oncoming cars and bikes and they can see you. Always assume they can't see you.

WHAT TO DO WHEN YOU HAVE
A BAD RUN OR RACE

BAD RUNS AND RACES WILL HAPPEN many, many times, but you will be stronger for it. My worst race was the Tokyo Marathon in 2015. I traveled to Japan for the first time for the marathon with my mom and my uncle Jorge. To say that I trained for this race is an understatement. The Tokyo Marathon is late February, so I logged 20-mile training runs over the icy streets of Manhattan to make this race happen. I wasn't just trying to complete 26.2 miles, I was trying to slay the shit out of this race and my PR to qualify for the Boston Marathon. I built it up so much in my mind that I might as well have made it a holiday. Best-laid plans . . .

Tokyo is a wonderland of oddity, fashion, and insane vibes—my kind of city. The energy on race day was no different. However, while cruising through mile 13, I heard an alarm. It was my insulin pod failing, which, as a type-one diabetic, I need not only to run but also to live. I immediately knew I was fucked. I wasn't running with any spare insulin or a replacement pod. What did this mean for my body? Basically, my blood sugar levels will start to rise with no insulin and I risk ketosis, which means my body becomes acidic. People can end up in the hospital with ketosis. It's not cute. Even with insulin, I do a delicate dance on race day to combat high highs and low lows. In this moment, when my pod failed, my blood sugar was at 175—I normally aim for 90–100—which is high, but not alarming. You need fuel to race, but fuel was going to make my blood sugar rise even higher so I didn't consume any food, only water.

Have you heard of hitting the wall during a race? It often occurs during mile 21 of a marathon, when your body is fatigued and you don't have enough fuel, energy, or physical ability to continue. I basically finished this race with a

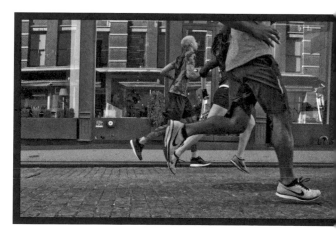

self-induced deficit of fuel just so I could avoid ketosis and cross the finish line. Runners who hit the wall know that feeling all too well of willing a single, solitary step of forward momentum. By mile 16 I was feeling fatigue, way too early for a race I trained this well for, but I would not stop. By mile 19 I was delirious and running a solid 2 minutes per mile slower than my race pace. By mile 22 I was praying; legit side-of-the-road, God-take-me-now praying, and I cried a little. And then I decided to finish the damn thing. I crossed the finish in 3:55.

I was deeply disappointed about that race for a while. Not only was my time far from a personal record, but I'd never felt that weak before and it was terrifying. It sent me into a gnarly mental place until I realized that because of it I would forever run smarter (aka carrying extra insulin on me) and stronger. I sincerely hope you never have a run like that, but if you do, just know that you are a boss and it will only make you stronger. It's just a road.

THREE WAYS TO COPE WITH A SHITTY RUN

1

Grieve it.
It's okay to mourn a terrible race when your hopes were high, but don't indulge this feeling for more than a few days. If you're brooding over a terrible training run, remember that a bad training run is better than a bad race day, and it's the bad training runs that sometimes help make our best races.

2

Celebrate it.
Seriously. You're going to be smarter and stronger because of it. What could you have done differently? Did you start too fast? Undertrain? Underfuel? Dissect it with someone you trust (it helps to talk about it). Learn from it, and then move on.

3

Sign up for another race.
There's always another finish line on the horizon. Dust yourself off and set your sights high. It's important to think of this race as an entirely separate event, *not* a do-over of the bad one. If you're still feeling angry or desperate to prove something, space out the next race to give yourself time to recover.

SUCCESS
FEELS
SWEETER
WHEN IT'S
EARNED.
MAKE
YOURS
TASTY.

GETTING STRONGER INVOLVES STANDING STILL.

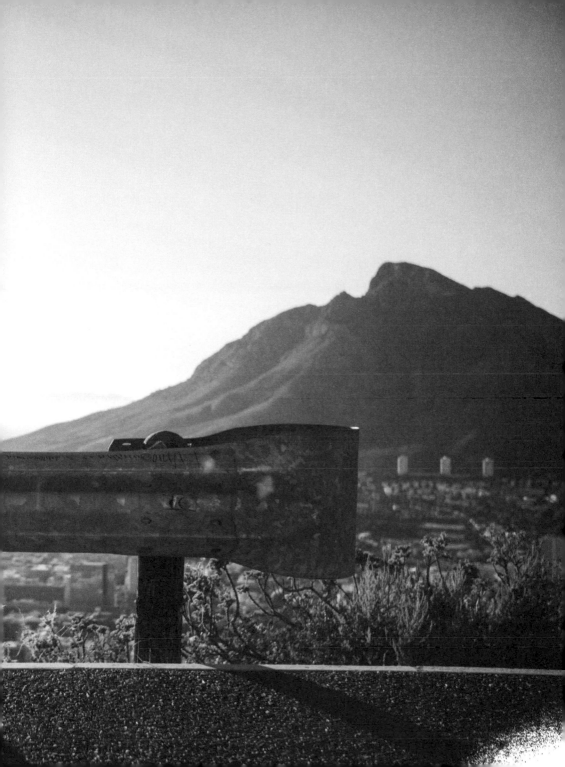

NINE POSTRACE RECOVERY TIPS

IF YOU'RE COMING OFF A RACE, especially any race lasting longer than 90 minutes, try these nine tips to heal faster and get back out there.

1. **Rest.** Once you get in a running groove, you might want to do it every day, all the time. If that sounds crazy, trust me, you might get there. I did. Rest is actually much harder for me to accomplish than a tough workout. At least one day a workout cycle should be devoted to rest, especially if you have a race coming up or just finished one. Common advice is once a week, but I know plenty of ultramarathon runners who rest on a ten-day or two-week or even a month-long cycle.

2. **Listen to your body** and err on the side of resting if you're not sure. Overtraining leads to injury. Injuries are not cute.

3. **Ice everything,** especially if it hurts, but even if it doesn't hurt. If I had to choose between icing and stretching, ice would win. The ice packs that are used for food deliveries like Blue Apron are awesome to use for ice baths. After a race, I ice my knees, quads, and my feet. Twenty minutes on, 20 minutes off, repeat.

4. **Arnica gel** is great for pain relief. Massage it on your calves and sole arches.

5. **Move.** It's counterintuitive, but unless you're injured you should at least walk the day after a race. Don't get turned up with miles for at least two weeks, though.

6. **Fuel with anti-inflammatory foods** such as ginger, cherries, beets, dark leafy greens, and foods rich in omega-3 like walnuts. Foods high in artificial sugar and saturated fat can increase inflammation.

7. **Elevate your feet.** Sit in an L shape with your back on the floor or couch, and your feet above you against a wall. It really helps prevent swelling.

8. **Spin.** I've coached indoor cycling within a day or two of racing and I swear the cross-training, low-impact movement, and endorphins of spinning help with recovery.

9. **Sleep. Like. A. Mofo.** Nothing beats the human growth hormone that releases while you sleep to help repair muscle tissue.

TAPER MODE

TAPERING means easing up on training leading up to race day. This period can last as little as a few days before a race to as much as three weeks. The shorter the distance, the shorter the taper.

Before a marathon, I'm in that sitting-in-the-park-drinking-ginger-juice mode. It's hard to hold back when you're ready to rock. I actually hate to taper and have a hard time listening to my better judgment and sitting the hell down.

The taper crazies are real. You've spent months leading up to one race and ideally you reach the taper period like a caged racehorse.

For a marathon taper, I recommend reducing mileage three weeks from race day by 20–25 percent of total weekly mileage. While most of your miles during this time should feel easy, effort sessions are essential during this period, too. It doesn't mean just sit back and slow down. If you have a goal pace, log 5–6 miles a week until race day at that pace.

Two weeks out, reduce by another 25 percent. Doubt tends to creep in during this time and you think about training you could have or should have done. Tough love. It's too late to make any gains so meet your body where it is. A solid leg refresher during taper week two is a 2-mile repeat session 30 seconds faster (no more) than your goal race pace.

Race week is about sleep and nourishment. There's literally nothing you can do to get faster or better in the days leading up to a race, but you can exhaust your mind and body. Run 3–4 times this week at a light pace. The purpose of these runs is to maintain blood volume that you've built up during training and to stay sane! Experienced marathoners with a time goal should do sharpening sessions of 1–4 miles at race pace and a shakeout run the day before of 1–2 miles at an easy pace.

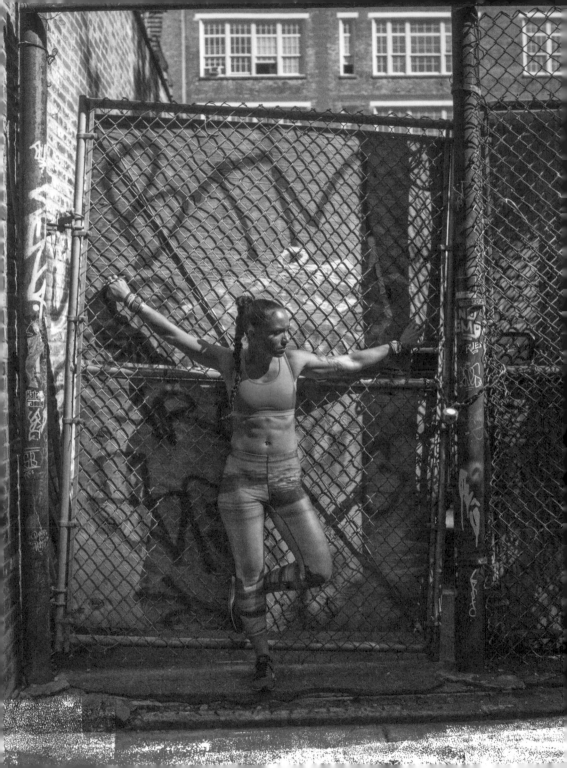

MY FIVE RACE DAY TAPER TIPS

1. **Nothing new on race day.** This includes food, gear, and your race T-shirt. Start thinking about what you've used to fuel during training runs. You'll want to eat the same foods that have worked already. No need to test out a new Gu Energy Gel or PowerBar on race morning and risk an upset stomach. The testing phase should happen long before race day.

2. **Now is not the time** to try yoga, barre, Pilates, or any other workout for the first time. If you're a regular yogi and you know a yoga session will keep you limber, not sore or injured, go for it. But *nothing* new.

3. **Trust the training.** Nerves are normal, but as race day approaches and doubts slip through the cracks, remember that no single workout from now until race day will make or break your race.

4. **Listen to your body.** Your eating habits may have changed with the increased demands of training. As your mileage decreases until race day (about 20 percent of mileage a week), remember to eat when you are hungry, not just because you've made a habit of meals before or after training runs. Ten-milers don't require the same fuel as four-milers.

5. **Not running can feel like torture.** Your brain goes wild thinking about what you should or shouldn't have done in terms of training. Use this extra time to catch up with loved ones, watch that movie you've been wanting to see, or read that book. Savor it!

DEALING WITH POSTRACE BLUES

POSTRACE BLUES ARE A TRUE OCCURRENCE. You've built up the race for months, driven your family and friends crazy with this preoccupation, and whether it was a wonderful race or a tough one, it's common to feel "meh" in the days that follow after you cross the finish line. Not only has your body been tested, but your emotions, serotonin, and endorphins have surged. Of course your body's going to be like, "What the F?!" after it. The important thing is learning how to deal with the postrace blues.

- **It's okay if you have no desire to run.** As your body recovers, now is a great time to ease into the cross-training that you neglected while preparing for the race. Maybe look into a new sport such as swimming or cycling.

- **Sign up for another race of a different distance.** If you raced a 5K, consider a mud run or an adventure race series like Spartan. If you conquered a marathon, try a local 10K for speed or an ultra for distance. This will force you to shift gears and get out of the pace and training mode for the race you just finished.

- **Visualization that works for race day works now, too.** See yourself getting out the door for a chill 30-minute run. See yourself lacing up. Tell yourself you're only going for 10 minutes; once you get started you'll likely do a longer run. Track your first recovery run in minutes, not miles. No watch. Even if you don't feel sore, your body has been through a lot.

- **The buddy system matters now more than ever.** If you've never run with a group or a friend, start now. It's a wonderful opportunity to get those negative vibes out of your system with someone who likely empathizes. Check out Meetup.com or local running stores for group run options.

- **Write it out!** If you simply can't muster energy to get off the couch, write down how you feel. No joke, it's cathartic.

If you're concerned that your postrace blues are serious, don't hesitate to see a medical professional. Better safe than sorry!

MORE RECOVERY VIBES

BESIDES THE INITIAL postrace recovery tips on page 114, here are more advanced ones.

- A massage is glorious for sore muscles, but wait at least twenty-four hours before jumping on the massage table. Manipulating muscles that are too sore can do more harm than good. The massage tents at the end of races know how sore you might be and are generally mindful of this. Tell them if it's too much!

- A foam roller and the Marathon Stick are great for self-myofascial release. Both of these tools work by rolling knots out of muscles and relieving muscle tightness. Consistency is key. Using them for only five-minutes the day after a race isn't enough to break up fascia and flush out the buildup of lactic acid in your legs caused by running. Consistent rolling after every run is ideal. After a race or long run, roll for 5 minutes, lingering on tight spots. If you're in severe pain or too tender, skip that spot and revisit it during the next foam-rolling session. Let me be clear, though: foam rolling will hurt at times, so don't expect it to feel good. These tools can be purchased online or at your local sporting goods store.

- Sit with your back down on the floor or couch and prop your legs up against a wall in an L-shape position to get the blood flowing in the opposite direction. Hold this for 5–7 minutes. Do this every day the week after the race before bed and your body will thank you. Breathe in deep, calming breaths while you're doing it. The more you can relax into the pose the better.

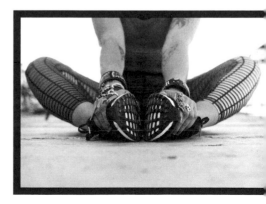

- Above all else, ice, ice, baby. Ice is always a good idea. Ice baths are thought to reduce inflammation and muscle soreness caused by intense, repetitive exercise.

LETTING GO

CREATES SPACE FOR GOOD THINGS TO HAPPEN.

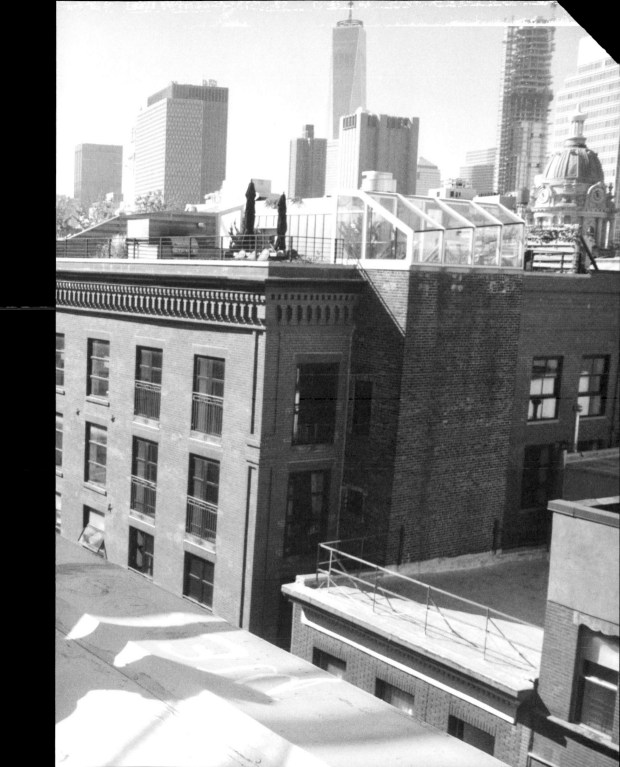

HOW TO TAKE AN ICE BATH

1. Consider being conservative with how cold you go for your first plunge. I would start at 55 degrees Fahrenheit and get colder as you go.

2. Start with sitting in the water for 5 minutes, but definitely don't go over 10 minutes. Hypothermia is not cute so pay attention to the color of your toes. If they start to turn blue, get out!

3. Make a hot beverage to drink during the ice bath. If you don't drink coffee or tea, just sip some hot water with lemon. Having something hot in your hands distracts from the cold temps.

4. The first 2 minutes are the hardest. You will adjust. Put on the radio or a podcast. Do whatever it takes to distract you from the cold.

5. The ice packs that are used to keep coolers cold are great for ice baths. Keep them in your freezer. Do not use if any of the content is breaking through! That stuff is toxic.

6. Don't immediately jump into a hot shower when you're done. Wrap yourself up in a blanket and let the cold linger.

ICING AN INJURY

- Ice as soon as you feel the discomfort.

- Don't ice and then work out. Chilling your muscles before trying to move them is not a good idea.

- More is not better. Keep the ice for no longer than 20 minutes. Repeat 4–5 times a day with at least 30 minutes between each ice session.

- Consistency is key with icing and stretching. This is not a one-and-done affair.

- Cooling gel and arnica can also have an effect similar to icing. These are a good option when you're at work or just can't sit back with an ice pack.

SPRING TRAINING TIPS

GETTING OUT THERE for a run can be hard once the temperature starts to drop. I get it. But here is some real love advice for when the sun comes back to play.

1. Start where you're at, not where you *want* to be. This is essential for avoiding injury and unrealistic expectations. If you haven't been running for a few weeks or months, then your legs probably aren't prepared for a 5-mile run out the gate. That's okay. Be honest. Start with the first step, not what your PR was a year ago. You'll get back there.

2. Reassess you gear. Have you been running in the same shoes all year? It might be time for a fresh pair. Running stores often suggest a new pair after 300 miles. I think most running shoes can handle upwards of 500 miles. If you notice significant wear in the soles or decreased support in the arch, it's a sign that you need a new pair irrespective of how many miles you've run in them.

3. Reinforce your training pyramid. Training plans are a pyramid. Build your base now. Gradually increase your weekly mileage by 10 percent a week. For example, if you've been running once or twice a week for 30 minutes throughout the winter, take it to no more than 3–4 times a week for 30 minutes until you build your base. Once you have a base of easy miles, you can begin to build on your speed, stamina, and longer runs. Adding speed work too soon can risk injury. Go easy.

4. You can't out-train a bad diet. Eat like you love yourself. Fuel for greatness 80 percent of the time and the other 20 percent can be food porn.

5. Have you been training like a beast all winter? Then I salute you. Take advantage of your consistency and mix it up! It's a long road of summer training to fall marathons.

CHALLENGE: One of my favorite challenges is running 5K a day, every day, for one month. I started this in December 2014 to keep me running through the cold and now I'm challenging you. Choose a month and aim for a specific distance every day. The consistency is more of a challenge than the distance is. It's tough to get out every day, but you'll be stronger for it. Challenge your homies to join and hashtag social media posts with #3for31 (even if it's a short month).

VISUALIZATION TIP

FACING OUR FEARS HELPS US CONQUER THEM.
Visualizing how we will handle rough runs gives us a resource if the worst-case scenario actually occurs. Some common concerns are cramping, running alone, racing with others, blisters, hitting the wall, wardrobe malfunctions, and tummy trouble. Think about your worst possible racing or training scenario. Write down these fears, irrational or not, and how you will deal with them. Do NOT do this the night before race day because it might stress you out. Do this during training so you have time to try your solutions and allay your fears. It's never as bad in reality as it is in our heads.

LAUGHTER

IS THE
TRUE WAY
TO A
SIX-PACK.

"SET YOUR
LIFE ON FIRE.
SEEK THOSE
WHO FAN
YOUR FLAMES."
—RUMI

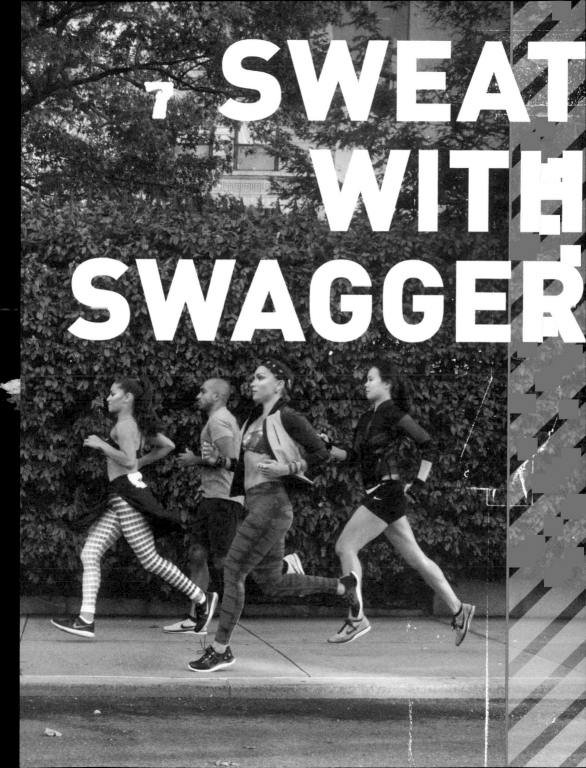

7 SWEAT WITH SWAGGER

SWEATING WITH SWAGGER IS ABOUT DOING YOU REGARDLESS OF WHAT OTHERS MIGHT THINK OR SAY.

IF YOU LOOK GOOD, YOU WILL FEEL GOOD AND WORK HARDER. Show up dressed for the job you want, right? If the job you want is to be a victorious athlete, then dress for victory.

Sweating with purpose, power, and swagger is the exclamation point behind a ferocious athlete. Those are the ones who don't sacrifice style for function. There's an amazing freedom that comes with knowing you're a runner even when you don't look like a runner.

The running gear that is sold can be daunting in its extent, and damn expensive. I'm not saying you should spend one month's rent on running gear. But once a season, you've earned a new pair of running shoes and at least one fly pair of tights, shorts, or a jacket to keep you soaring. I left law so spandex could be business casual and I'm marinating in it! "Sweat with swagger" is my ethos. It's not just a visual conversation we are having with the world, but a lived aesthetic.

Swagger is a lifestyle choice. We don't need to wake up every morning with a spring in our step to do things that stoke the fire in our bellies. Sometimes there are days where you have to fake it till you make it. Then before you know it, you're strolling down the street like it's a runway and running the track like it's a catwalk.

I showed up to my first 50-mile ultramarathon, the North Face Endurance Challenge in Washington, D.C., with zero clue of what I was doing and I was ill-prepared. I had no water, a headlamp, and four-finger gold rings. Guess what? I got it done on my terms. Yes, there are practical necessities (I now always bring water on a trail ultra), but there's a moment when we are suiting up to run that it feels like we are putting on armor. My rings, my cat eyeliner, bandana, and red lipstick are *my* superhero gear. Maybe yours is a photo of your kid pinned to your shorts, an all-black race kit, or a goofy hat. Dance your dance, baby. If someone's too serious to respect something that inspires, motivates, and makes you move, then I have two letters for them, *FU*, and two words, *Lighten up!*

This chapter is all about stocking up your running arsenal with the gear you'll need to get up, get out, and start running. I love the simplicity of running. The ability to just shut up and run doesn't take much, but that doesn't mean you can't have fun with your gear. Bold prints and pops of color are staples for me. Running shoes and clothes are the skeleton and can be as practical as necessary; just remember there's a balance between practicality and fun. I've found leggings for five bucks on Manhattan's Canal Street that are a far cry from technical running tights. If it doesn't chafe and isn't see-through, it works for me. You don't have to wear gear strictly dubbed "running apparel" to make it work on a run.

Headbands, socks, waist packs, jewelry, and laces can get as crazy as you're comfortable with. Swapping out plain laces with colorful ones for otherwise bland shoes can give you a surprising boost. Guys, you can have fun, too. The road is our runway. Why not be bold with it? I always subscribe to the adage "do you." If all black and monochrome is your look, awesome. That's the entire point of sweating with swagger. If it doesn't feel good, leave it at home.

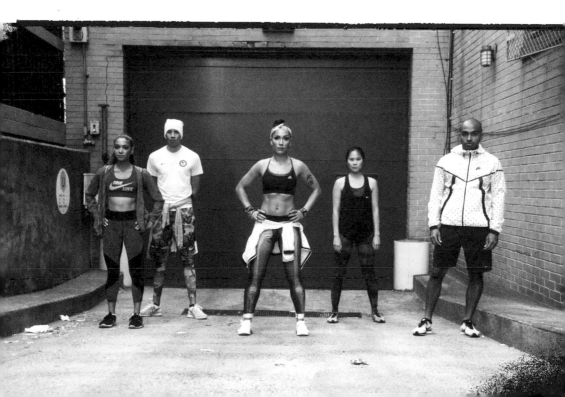

SWEAT IS
YOUR BEST
ACCESSORY.

NUMBER-ONE GEAR ESSENTIAL?
YOUR SHOES

KNOW I'VE SAID THIS BEFORE, but the most important piece of gear you need to run is a good pair of running shoes. This is not where you skimp on quality. Shoes absorb impact for thousands of steps. The same ones you need to hike, climb, stroll, or twerk are not necessarily the ones you need to run, race, and compete. Go to a local running store that performs a gait analysis of how you run. Finding the right shoes is like dating. It can take trial and error. Don't be afraid to return the shoes if they don't work after a few miles. Any legit running store will take an ill-fitting shoe back.

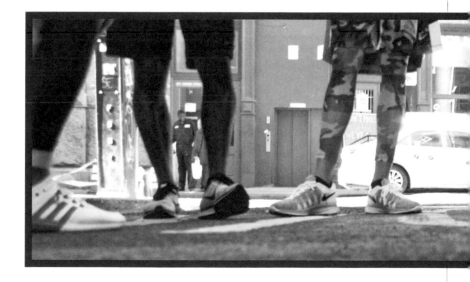

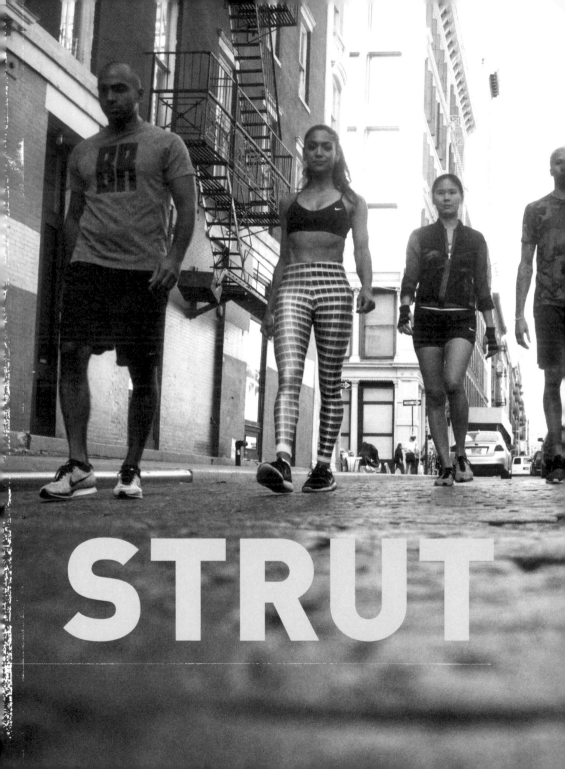

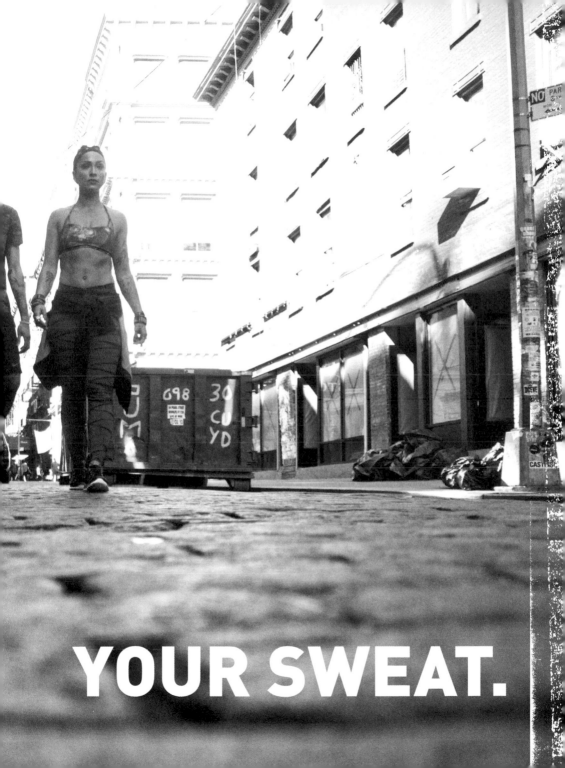

YOUR SWEAT.

STOCK UP YOUR RUNNING ARMORY

1. **Road ID:** I recommend ordering your own customized rubber Road ID bracelet, which lists essential information like your name, emergency contact, and allergy info. It allows you to run without an ID and, should there be an emergency, provides medics with the necessary information to give you the right care. Visit roadid.com.

2. **Foam roller:** A foam roller or the Marathon Stick you see at every marathon expo is a great way to loosen tight muscles from glutes to hamstrings to shoulders. I've spent many days just staring at the foam roller on my living room floor. You actually have to use it for it to work! I also have a tennis ball that I use under the arch of my feet. Put on an old episode of your favorite show and give your muscles some love.

3. **Running sleeves:** Dressing for weather can sometimes feel like such a fickle task. For early morning runs when the weather is cooler, arm sleeves are perfect. You can just roll them down when you warm up, and they give you mad super-hero status.

4. **Calf sleeves:** Compression gear in general is good to try for recovery. Calf sleeves can reduce swelling, but they can also be uncomfortable or ineffective for some. I love them and recommend you give them a try to see if they work for you. Zensah is my favorite brand.

5. **Essential oils:** This might seem random, but essential oils are amazing for motivation. I discovered that lemon and peppermint essential oils on my neck got me out during frigid winter runs. It also smells better than sweat. Scent is a powerful motivator, my friends.

6. **Chafe stick:** Sometimes the rubbing of skin involved in logging miles makes us chafe. Guys, I'm talking about bloody nipples. Ladies, under arms or inner thigh. There are various brands of chafe sticks out there that can alleviate this unpleasant side effect to training. Good old-fashioned petroleum jelly works, too.

7. **Kinesio Tex tape (KT tape):** Kinesio Tex tape is an elastic tape that can improve blood flow under the area where it's applied. Some runners put KT tape on their legs to help secure injured areas such as Achilles' tendons or iliotibial bands while they run. Some people swear by it and some, like me, have never used it.

WHAT HAVE YOU DONE TODAY TO FEEL PROUD?

WEATHER

WEATHER CAN BE A CHALLENGE when it comes to getting out for a run, especially cold weather. People tend to run at different temps. I can run in a sports bra and microscopic shorts well into a New York fall, while I have friends who have a thermal on in September. I recommend dressing for weather 10 degrees warmer than your phone app or the weather forecaster says because you're going to warm up a mile into your run. As with everything that applies to running, it's all trial and error. Find out what works for YOU.

SUMMER ESSENTIALS

1. **Water.** Hydration is key when you are sweating buckets. If you stop sweating, it's an indicator that you need to drink because you're dehydrated. If you're running in an area that doesn't have places to buy water or accessible drinking fountains, invest in a running hydration pack.

2. **Salt.** When you sweat you lose sodium in your body. Replacing the salt you lose is especially important on hot days. Most electrolyte tablets and drinks contain some sodium. If you're the type of runner who ends up with white salt deposits after a run, be super-mindful of this during long runs. Salt tablets might be a good option for you. One year during a hot New York City Marathon, I was cramping so bad that I stuck a salt packet from a bodega under my tongue. It was gross but did the trick.

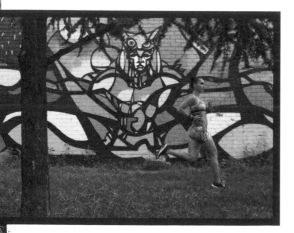

3. **Sweat-wicking gear.** Shorts and tops that wick sweat work by spreading out the moisture over the fabric so that it dries quickly. It's amazing for long, hot summer runs.

4. **Shades.** Squinting for any amount of time during a run actually wastes a ton of energy. Invest in a good pair of sunglasses that have a snug fit so they don't bounce on your face while you run.

WINTER ESSENTIALS

1. **Gloves and either earmuffs or a hat.** Two of the main places to retain heat and where you feel the cold are your hands and ears, so look into purchasing gloves and either earmuffs or a snug hat. I use cheap gloves from a dollar store for most of the fall season. Below-freezing temps might require thin, insulated running gloves and/or hand warmers.

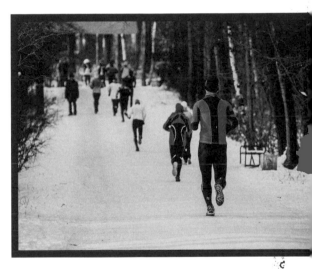

2. **Coconut oil and lip balm.** A windburned, chapped face is a real thing, people, and it sucks! Invest in lotion and lip balm to protect yourself against the cold winds while you run.

3. **Wick gear, or Under Armour.** Wick gear is even more important in the winter than in the summer. Sweat on cotton clothes is going to freeze. Any layer in direct contact with your skin needs to be a material that dries quickly and retains heat. Layers are a must.

4. **A Buff or bandana.** When the wind is whipping at your face, sometimes you need more than just lotion. I usually wrap a Buff or bandana around the lower half of my face to protect my skin from the cold. Add a few drops of essential oil for a lift.

MAKE IT YOURS

THERE'S NO BETTER FEELING than hearing a stranger call your name during a race. You feel like everyone is there to cheer you on. Roll out the red carpet and let the crowds sing your praises by writing your name on your shirt. You trained for this day. Own it by personalizing your gear.

What do you do with all those old race shirts? A pair of scissors and a glue gun go a long way. Get *Edward Scissorhands* on that shit. I love cutting the sleeves off old shirts and creating a fringe effect. I've even created minidresses from super-big ones. I customize most of my bras and almost all of my T-shirts. Any craft store sells letter decals. Buy a pack of one- or two-inch letters and iron them onto your race day T-shirt, sports bra, or shorts. Remember to wear the shirt before race day to make sure it doesn't chafe or itch.

During the race expo, don't buy a bunch of new shit. You'll be temped to wear it or use it on race day and there's not enough time to test new gear. Nerves and a race day expo are *not* a good combo. Pick up your bib and bounce. I know it's tempting to try the brand-new shoes, watch, shirt, gel, massage, but step away. Check out an expo when you're *not* racing. That's the time to experiment with new gear.

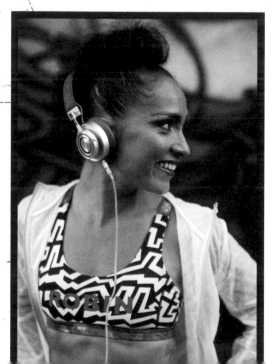

YOUR
PHOTO
HERE

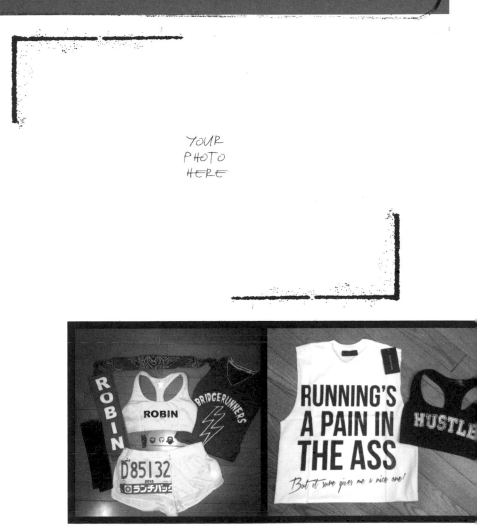

YOU ONLY
REGRET THE
RUN YOU
DIDN'T DO.

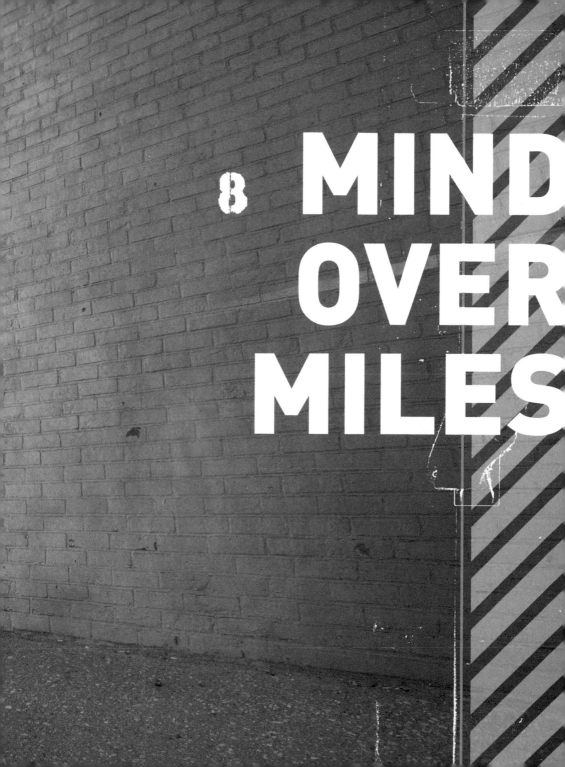

8 MIND OVER MILES

HEAD GAMES

YOU ARE NOT YOUR THOUGHTS, yet everything we are is a result of our thinking. When we take responsibility for our thoughts and perceptions, the running game becomes ours. When it comes to training, your mind is the most powerful tool. Period.

Most of us are stuck in various habituated, reactive, and conditioned thinking patterns. It is important to recognize the thought forms that constrict our perception, thinking, feeling, and acting. How do we do this?

Pushing the pause button to focus our attention inward requires one thing—mindful breathing, or meditation. It's a simple concept in theory but can be difficult in practice. In creating change, most experts agree that it takes at least 66 days to cement any behavior. Developing a daily conscious control of the mind is essential for every athlete and attainable through the practice of mindfulness.

The word *mindfulness* is thrown around a lot. I describe it as nonjudgmental awareness of the mind's contents on a moment-to-moment basis. Our runs are nothing but footsteps, thoughts, moments, and sweat. When we take the wheel of our fast-acting, negative thought patterns, we run on a whole new playing field.

Think of meditation as push-ups for your brain. One push-up does not create core strength. Consistent push-ups create champions. There are many meditation traditions such as Vipassana, Vedic, Transcendental, and every combination of the three going back to Buddha. Whatever your entry point, there's a "right" way to do it as long you can stick with it.

I started my meditation practice with Gabrielle Bernstein meditations. Initially, I had no attention span. For more than a year, my meditation efforts were peppered with questions: Am I doing this right? Is this meditation? What if I can't stop thinking? I learned through frustration and pauses that meditation is really about breathing with intention.

Ultramarathons have taught me the art of visualization and mindfulness, and sports psychologists and spiritual leaders alike know the power of the mind. Not only can meditation change your brain matter, but it can also alleviate stress, anxiety, and the pervasive mind chatter we all battle.

Trust me, I'm no Zen master. I still curse like a trucker, lose my cool, and have irrationally negative thoughts. Meditation is called a practice for a reason.

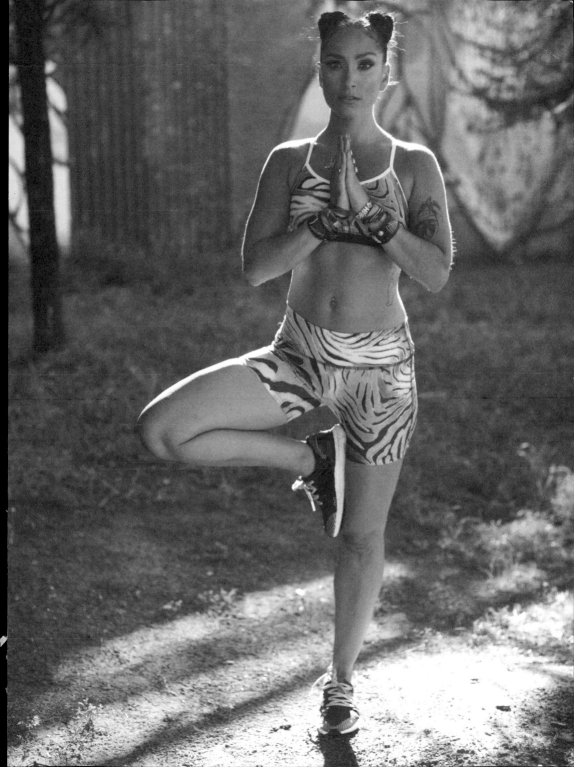

TEN NEWBIE MEDITATION TIPS

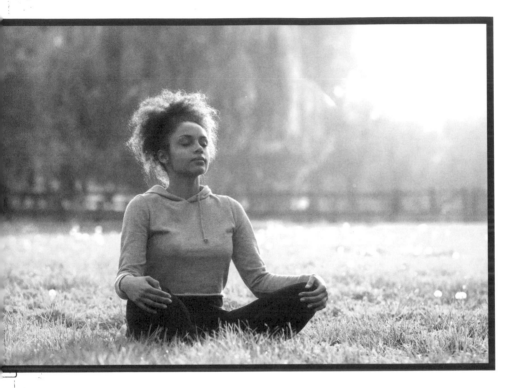

1. **Do YOU and Experiment.** There's no "wrong" way to meditate. It's all about establishing consistency and rhythm. There are so many different types of teachers, methods, and online communities to help you along your journey. Music? Religious conversations? Mantras? Walking meditation? Candle meditation? TM? Vedic? Do some research and see what works. There are as many styles of meditation as there are meditators.

2. **Guided Meditation.** I love Gabrielle Bernstein guided meditations. They are only 5–6 minutes, which helped me start because I didn't feel like I was devoting too much time. Apps like Simply Being are also recommended for guided focus. You can select 5–20 minute nature sounds, music, or a spoken guide.

3. **Commit to 66 Days.** Studies show that doing something consistently for 66 days reinforces habit. Mindfulness is a practice and getting into the habit of waking up and meditating helped me stay consistent. If you fall off, there's always tomorrow.

4. **Start Small.** Take a few minutes out of your day to meditate. Maybe you'll be able to dive right into hour-long meditations. If not, I suggest starting small; take three minutes to walk and concentrate on your breathing.

5. **Don't Stress About It.** I've had many stops and starts with meditation. My inner monologue was often abuzz with questions and random thoughts: Am I doing this right? What am I having for lunch? What do I need to do today? For me, meditation is not about nothingness; it's about acknowledging what pops up in my head at the time and clearing my internal channel. I've really found this to be a powerful tool in manifesting my passions and desires, and helping to motivate me.

6. **Breathe.** I have mini-meditations all the time. Breathe in for four counts, hold it for four, and then release for four. I literally do this whenever I find myself getting impatient, stressed, or negative. It's a practice used by the military to steady soldiers before battle. Powerful shit!

7. **Let It Go.** Some days will be better than others. Don't focus on daily practice! Just do the best you can every day, and then let it go.

8. **Start the Day Off with Meditation.** Meditating first thing in the morning helped me establish it as a practice as well as put me in a peaceful state of mind at the start of the day. It also helped for me to do it before grabbing my phone to check emails, tweets, Instagram likes, etc. Silence the noise. We can't be tuned in every second of the day.

9. **Fake It Till You Make It.** You might feel silly at first. I did. However, I found that going through the motions actually allowed me to believe in the breathing and mantras.

10. **Dwell in Possibility.** You can only have in your life what you believe is possible. For real! Meditation helps quiet the mind. Every day you have a choice to be your most giving, loving, powerful self. Do not resist the mind directly; befriend it and make it your companion. Gradually, expand your attention span by small increments over time.

NAMASTE, MY PEOPLES.

THE USE OF MANTRAS

I NOW PRACTICE a mantra-based meditation practice in the Vedic tradition. My teacher, Ben Turshen, is also a former lawyer turned athlete. I learned this tradition from him and it stuck. *Mantra* is Sanskrit for "instrument for thinking." Short words or phrases have long been used to focus the mind in meditation. In the Vedic tradition, a mantra is assigned from the teacher to the student and never uttered aloud. My meditation mantra is different than my motivational mantra when I'm running. Play with what works for you. Olympic marathoner and running coach Jeff Galloway coined "RPG" as his mantra, which stands for "relax, power, glide." Short mantras of two to three words work well.

MY MANTRA IS "I AM."

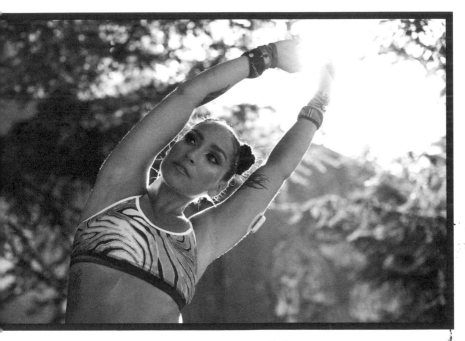

CREATE YOUR OWN MANTRA

I want you to develop your own running mantra. Keep it short and positive. Instead of "This hurts" think "This is progress. I'm closer." A good mantra diverts your mind from thoughts that reinforce the pain to thoughts that help you transcend it. It doesn't matter if it's just a combination of words, or gibberish—it need only have meaning to you.

Choose one word from each category and play with creating different mantras below. On your next run, practice repeating this mantra. The more you associate emotion and movement with the mantra, the more powerful it becomes. This is not a one-and-done thing. Give it 5–10 runs to see if it sinks in. As with everything in this book, take what works and leave what doesn't.

1.	2.	3.	4.
Run	Strong	Think	Power
Go	Fast	Feel	Speed
Stride	Quick	Embrace	Brave
Sprint	Light	Be	Bold
Be	Fierce	Build	Courage
Move	Hard		Swagger

BREATHE

ONE OF THE MOST IMPORTANT ASPECTS of running and meditation is breathing. Learning how to properly take in and expel air will help you become a better runner. Oxygen is more than physiology. It's our body's natural destressor. There are effective ways to alleviate nerves as well as run more efficiently with breath control. Most people breathe with their chest rather than their bellies. Chest breathing is short, shallow breaths, and during a run wastes energy. Belly breathing is defined as deep breathing. The lungs take in more air so that not only do they expand but your belly does as well (hence the name belly breathing). So, how do you tell the difference?

First, take a deep breath with your mouth open. Relax your face. On the exhale, release the tension. On the next inhale, concentrate on filling your lungs completely and exhale through your back. Focus on your center—the area right behind your belly button. Think about inflating your belly as you would inflate a balloon with air. That's the focus of belly breathing.

BEFORE A RUN

An easy exercise you can use before a race, or even a meeting, is actually taught to the military before drills. It's called tactical breathing (breath in for four counts, hold for four counts, out for four counts; repeat).

Breathing calms our neurological system. Similarly, whether you're running, lifting, or practicing yoga, breath carries oxygen to your muscles and propels your movement. You don't need to be a yogi to benefit from this innate stress reliever.

HOW TO RELAX THE BODY WHILE RUNNING

1. **Cadence breathing:** When you inhale for two steps and exhale for one. If this feels too labored, start with a 5-count (inhale for 3 and exhale for 2). While you're focusing on breath work, it's best to leave the headphones at home. Tuning in to your breath is one of the best things you can do to understand your body's natural cadence and, eventually, your race pace.

2. **Refocus:** When you're running, do a head-to-toe body check. Relax your face and your shoulders. Are you clenching your hands? Your core? How's your form? Visualize strings pulling your legs up. Knees up. Light landing.

3. **Arm shake:** Every five minutes, completely loosen the shoulders, straighten the arms, and allow both arms to hang and wobble at your sides for 30 seconds as you run monkey-style.

4. **Tongue-press:** After the arm shake, press your tongue firmly against the roof of your mouth and hold it there for 8–10 seconds. Then allow it to relax, and as you do so, feel the tension release from your jaw and neck muscles. Focus on maintaining this relaxed jaw until your next tongue-press.

5. **Horizon-glance:** Pick a distant spot on the horizon and gaze at it for eight-ten seconds. This will encourage forward momentum and prevent too much time looking down at your feet or the road.

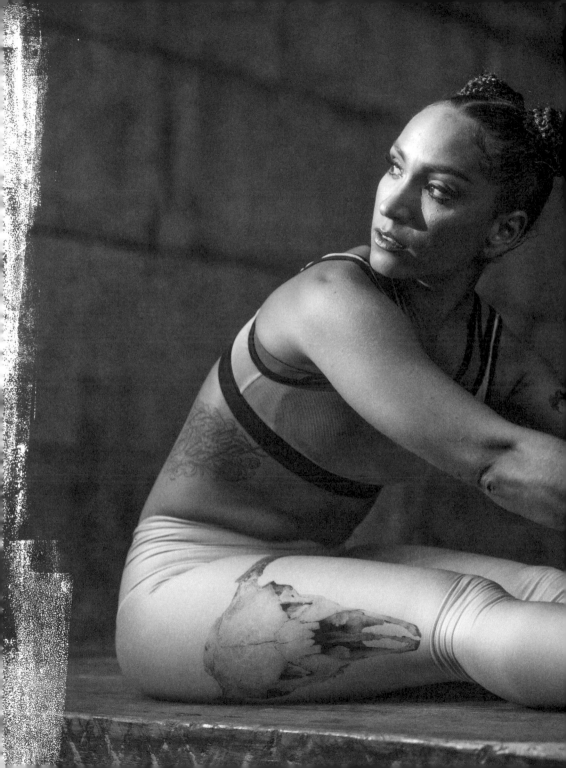

AFTER A RUN

AFTER A RUN, I recommend stretching, focusing on your breathing, and visualizing. If you had a bad run, breathe it out. If you had a great run, marinate in those vibes. Either way breath work will help your heart rate come down and allow your body to relax.

Belly breathing is ideal for relaxation. Lie down flat on your back. Place one hand on your belly and the other over your heart. Visualize your shoulders melting away from your ears. Allow your belly button to move in toward your spine. Breathe in for a count of 10, and then out for a count of 10. This is a great time to practice focusing on visualizations used on race day.

SURROUND YOURSELF WITH INSPIRATION

WILLPOWER IS A MUSCLE THAT FATIGUES, but it can also get stronger. You need to surround yourself with inspiration when you fall off your game. Whether you're diving into this book, an inspirational Tumblr, or calling a friend that just ran 13.1 miles—dig in.

INSPIRATION TIPS

- Put an inspirational note on your phone, your mirror, or at your desk. On it, include words and imagery that speak to you. It might seem cheesy at first, but the mind responds to visual cues.

- Change the title of your cell phone alarm to your mantra, or a saying like "Get it done" or "Do epic shit." That way you'll be inspired the minute you wake up.

- Rip out a page from a book if it speaks to you or print out a quote that inspires you. Put it up somewhere that is visible to you every day.

- And, as always, fake it till you make it!

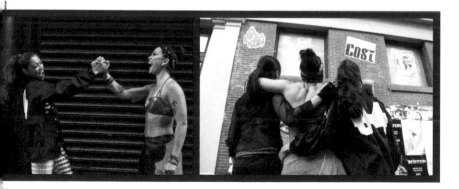

I WAS MADE TO ROAR AND SO ARE YOU.

SELF-TALK AND RACE DAY NERVES

WE HAVE APPROXIMATELY 60,000 THOUGHTS A DAY and, when we listen to our inner monologue, sometimes those thoughts can surprise us. It's a habitual conversation that most of the time we don't even realize we are having.

Our internal transcript can get loud before an important training run or race. The most effective way I've discovered to deal with race day nerves is belly breathing and free writing. Feeling both excited and nervous is healthy, and the adrenaline will get you to move. However, too much can be debilitating when we are repetitively playing out fears in our minds. Since we already addressed belly breathing, here are my tips for free writing—aka my brain dump.

Free writing is all about conceptualizing your concerns. Writing them down strips them of their power. Grab a pen and paper. Set a timer for 5 minutes of free writing, then write down everything on your mind related to your goal. This includes what you're excited about, what concerns you, and your fears, without a filter. Let it all flow onto the page. Nobody will read this (unless you want them to). No self-editing, no reservations. Be sure to write for the full 5 minutes even if you're writing, "What am I writing?"

After the 5 minutes, cross out what's out of your control. Circle anything positive and draw a box around concerns you can control. On a fresh page, list the positive feelings and then write out a game plan for race day addressing the concerns you put in a box. Playing out your race allows you to develop strategies to cope with stressors. If the situation arises, you will have rehearsed it in your mind and know how to deal with it.

Also, detailing a game plan starting from when you lay out your clothes to your racing strategy will address many practical concerns. The ones that linger are often out of our control. This is when you practice the art of letting go. The trick to managing negative thoughts is recognizing that you have the power to silence them. Your job is to focus on the positive list and the things you can control. Go to work.

VISUALIZATION TIP

DEVELOP YOUR RACE DAY SCRIPT.

- Picture your running shoes. Put them on. What are you wearing?
- Picture a running route that you enjoy or the race day course.
- You tell yourself to get going, to wake up; you have the ability to race so get out there . . . You are now feeling pumped, ready to compete at an optimal level.
- You're gliding. You start to feel your heart beating faster . . .
- See your knees come up high toward your chest and your heels extend behind you as you run quickly and smoothly; your heart is beating fast and your arms are pumping . . .
- Pay attention to your breathing. Notice how your muscles feel. You are feeling a sense of excitement and anticipation within yourself, yet you feel calm and in control.
- When you feel very fatigued, both physically and mentally, imagine yourself overcoming these feelings and giving your full effort.
- See yourself pick up the pace. Notice how your mood lifts and you observe more of your surroundings.
- Who is cheering you on from the sidelines? Is there music playing? Do you see anyone you know?
- Visualize the volunteers. They believe in you.
- You see yourself nearing the finish. What mile marker is it? Envision the finish.
- You focus on directing more power and strength to your legs. Your arms are pumping.
- Picture the medal. Run toward it. Feel the weight of the medal around your neck.
- Focus on your breath. Breathe deeply in through your nose. Out through your mouth. Breathe in strength. Breathe out doubt.
- As you breathe in, think "I." As you breathe out, think, "AM." I AM. I AM. Chant this internally as you cross the finish line.
- Slowly begin to come back to the present.

CREATE YOUR MENTAL "MOVIE REEL"

VISUALIZATION is a tried-and-true training technique that involves nothing more than seeing your success (aka crossing the finish line). When I interviewed Olympian Sanya Richards-Ross about her preparation for the London 2012 Games, she told me she watched videos of her track practices and created strategic mental movies. She then mentally rehearsed her 400 meters and visualized running the 400-meter race hundreds of times, in every lane on the track, against every competitor, before she even set foot in London.

We can use visualization to focus on specific movements/sport skills, specific outcomes, personal records, overcoming a difficult situation (cramping/weather), and regulating emotions (nerves).

While prepping for race day, I recommend creating a mental "movie" reel of your strongest training moments. Then replay it every night before you sleep or when you have a quiet moment.

To create a mental movie reel, spend 5 minutes recalling a positive race, run, mile, or experience related to your performance, even if it's unrelated to the sport. Do you remember an epic win in high school? It counts. I want you to write down two to three scenes for your movie reel, which should involve all the senses and be as detailed as possible. Where is the race? What do you see? What do you hear? What do you feel? Go a little deeper. What do you smell? Play around with this image of yourself. See yourself performing at your very best. Give yourself permission to dream, to push your current boundaries.

Once you have the images in your mind, close your eyes and watch your movie. Trace the movement of the breath as it enters and leaves your body. If possible, follow it all the way to your belly, and then back up, releasing any tension as it goes. With each breath, you relax a little more. You are breathing in strength and breathing out negativity. Feel the power in your body and the confidence in your voice. Bring your senses into the experience. Recall your movie moments. When you imagine yourself crossing the finish, feel the pride you'd feel with the medal around your neck.

Recap for Race Day
Before you start the race, bring up your mental movie reel. When you saw yourself performing, what was the vision of yourself like? Was it as though you were watching yourself on a TV screen, essentially seeing your entire body as well as everything around you, or was it more like you were looking out from your eyes, seeing things exactly as you would if you were there for real? Was it in color or black and white? The more we play with the movie and manipulate the mind, the better we get at visualization. Remember, these techniques are push-ups for the brain.

9

FUEL YOUR FIRE

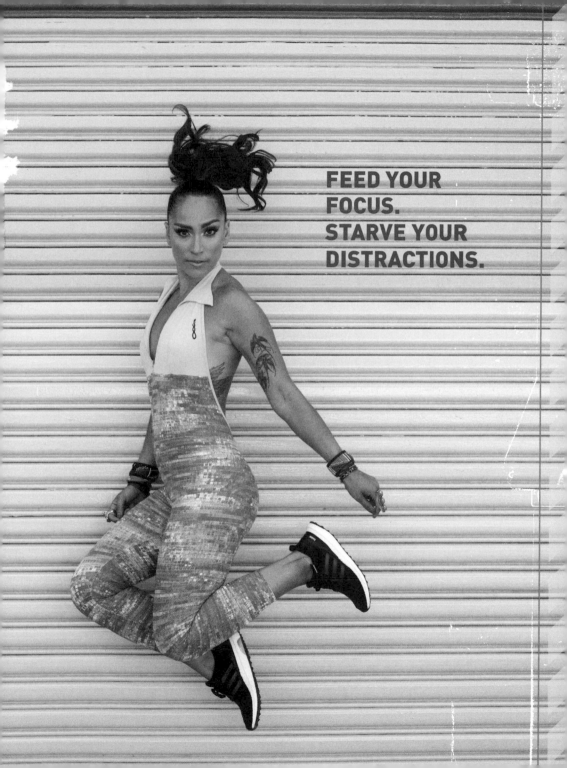

FEED YOUR
FOCUS.
STARVE YOUR
DISTRACTIONS.

WE'VE ALL HEARD IT.

What we consume directly affects how we feel and how our body performs. And I'm here to tell you it's true.

FACT:

Food can change you on a cellular level and what you eat affects how you run. Ultimately, what works for you when you run will be discovered through trial and error. Gastric issues are a longtime joke among runners. We push our bodies to the limit and our tummies sometimes suffer the consequence. However, eventually you develop a pre- and post-run eating regime that works for you.

I'M NOT A NUTRITIONIST. I EAT A LOT AND I RUN A LOT. HERE'S MY ADVICE:

As a rule of thumb, you want to consume 200 calories no later than 60 minutes before a run. Carbs give you energy and break down first. Not all carbs are created equal, so high-sugar pastries are not going to fuel you as efficiently or break down as evenly (from a glycemic perspective) as whole grains with a little protein. Generally, runners need 30–60 grams of carbs each hour they are running longer than 75 minutes.

THE 80/20 RULE

I DRINK MORE CHAMPAGNE THAN IS HUMANLY POSSIBLE; I love it! Literally, at Burning Man, a community festival in Nevada every August, I drink a bottle of champagne before most of my campmates wake up. I'm totally okay with this. Eighty percent of my life is healthy, driven, and balanced, while 20 percent is off-the-charts, pizza-in-my-face, hell-in-a-handbasket. The 80/20 Rule is basically being responsible for your body 80 percent of the time and just living during the other 20 percent. I'm not saying dabble in addictive and destructive drugs, but you should be able to eat a jar of Speculoos Cookie Butter from Trader Joe's every once in a while without hating yourself (add this food to the list of things that cannot enter my apartment because I have no self-control).

I didn't run my first mile until I was twenty-three. Because I never explored sports as a child, the last decade has been an adventure in pushing boundaries and engaging in the most important dialogue I've ever had with my body. It's self-evident that training and food power performance. The trial and error of finding the peak of performance changes as our bodies do.

Whether I'm preparing for a marathon, teaching three spin classes in a row, or running 150 miles in one week, the only constant is adaptation, meaning I have to listen to what my body is telling me. I don't eat meat, but I would never be prescriptive in nutrition advice. I share my fuel tips as a point of reference. It works for me and I hope you find what works for you.

It's not overly complicated. Stop eating crap. Seriously, I'm not a nutritionist, but think about how you want to perform and how you want to feel. It's not at the bottom of a bag of Cheetos. Trust me. If you can't pronounce the ingredients, put that shit down.

RUNNING WITH TYPE 1 DIABETES

I'M A TYPE 1 DIABETIC. That means my pancreas stopped producing insulin one day and I need insulin to live. It mostly sucks. I was diagnosed as an adult at the age of thirty-two, after a month-long trip to India. I felt really dehydrated, got blood work at my mom's urging, and boom, I need insulin forever. There's no known cause. Approximately 90 percent of adult diabetics are type 2, which is generally caused by lifestyle factors such as activity level and food choices. No matter what kind of diabetic you are, I want you to know something: you're a fucking bad-ass.

My immediate thought when I was diagnosed was, How can I continue to run ultras? I then remembered my friend Stephen England, who is a very accomplished marathoner, ultrarunner, and fellow type 1 diabetic (since the age of fourteen). Knowing he slayed the Leadville Trail 100 Run and other 100-milers was encouraging. I decided I was going to be unstoppable.

Running with diabetes hasn't always been pretty. It's been trial and error every single day. Within ten days of my diagnosis, I had all the technology available to assist with diabetes management. I use an OmniPod insulin pump (the white box on my arm or waist you see in photos) and a Dexcom glucose monitor, which alerts me to my blood glucose numbers. I firmly believe technology has kept me racing. I can adjust my insulin ratios for training, especially marathons and 3–4 hour long runs, without needing to inject insulin manually. More knowledge is power.

TIPS FOR INSULIN-DEPENDENT DIABETICS

1. **Everyone is different,** but I like to reduce my insulin slightly before a long run. I can run with 50–70 percent less insulin during a marathon. You have to see what works for you.

2. **Always carry something with sugar.** Fortunately, races normally have sports drinks laden with sugar (the only benefit!). I also stuff clementines in my race pack on long runs. I find them to be the perfect amount of sugar to keep me level without spiking.

3. **Love yourself anyway.** I've attempted 20-mile runs without pause and been sidelined by 3-mile runs for no reason. Many factors affect insulin and glucose levels. Love yourself anyway. No one training run will make or break a race.

4. **You might have high numbers after a race.** Adrenaline gets you to many finish lines. This can also cause spikes. Don't freak out. Weight lifting and boxing also make my blood sugars spike.

5. **This is controversial, but take your doctor's advice with a grain of salt.** I've had doctors who just don't understand what it means to race and commit to endurance sports with type 1 diabetes. They have suggested only eating carbs, and other super antiquated things related to food and movement. I'm no MD, so trust me, I understand how crazy this sounds, but, real talk: I know my body better than they do. And you probably do, too. Get your labs, take your sugars, know your A1C, but your gut rules everything. Bottom line: if you think you can do something, you probably can! I've always believed in superheroes. Some of us have insulin in our superhero belts. Don't let it stop you. Just run smart.

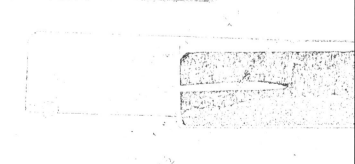

RUNS LESS THAN 60 MINUTES

IF YOU ATE PROPERLY THROUGHOUT THE DAY, you don't need to specifically fuel for a short run. If you must eat something before your sunrise session, I recommend the Rule of Half—half a banana, half a piece of toast with nut butter, half a protein bar. The Rule of Half is my standard for eating anything when it's less than 60 minutes before a run. Take in 200 calories and you should be good!

MY FAVORITE PRE-RUN SNACKS:
- Half an apple with almond butter
- A spoonful of peanut butter
- Half an avocado on rice toast
- Half a banana
- Half a pita or English muffin with cashew cheese (nondairy)
- Half a cup of coconut yogurt (or regular if you eat dairy) with berries, flax, and cinnamon

FUELING FOR MORNING RUNS

Early morning sessions can be done without fuel. In my experience, if I ate a decent dinner the night before I can perform a solid-effort session of 60 minutes or less on nothing more than water.

Hydration is the biggest thing people skimp on in the morning. You've been asleep for a number of hours without water. Dehydration makes you sluggish and cranky. I suggest a glass of hot water with lemon to start the day. Sip, don't chug. Chugging water and then running might lead to uncomfortable bloating.

If you're a coffee person, imbibe at least 30 minutes before your run. If you must eat something before your sunrise session, go with food that isn't greasy or loaded with fiber. Again, the Rule of Half is a good measure of how much food you need, and, of course, eat after your run! Within 30 minutes of your run, get in some carbs and protein.

THE EASY A.M. SHAKE

1 cup unsweetened almond milk
1 scoop protein (I use Vega protein,
   which is plant based)
½ banana (freeze them in halves so
   they are ready to go)
¼ cup berries (buy them frozen and
   organic)

Blend all ingredients together until
smooth. Feel free to add spinach and
other greens. You'll barely taste them,
plus they'll up your veggie game.

RUNS LONGER THAN 75–90 MINUTES

RUNS THAT ARE LONGER THAN 90 MINUTES ARE LONG RUNS. It doesn't matter if you're covering 6 miles or 15: it's a long enough time for your body to need more fuel. You need to train your gut and your palate to eat while running. You also need to discover what works for you. Runners' stomachs can be fickle as hell. What works for runners such as Meb Keflezighi or Kara Goucher might not work for you. You very well might not be the type of person who needs fuel on a 90-minute run, but you might also hit a wall. Get to know your needs by training with and without fuel. You definitely don't want to leave it to race day and try a new energy gel on the course.

If you're running longer than an hour, whether you feel it or not, your glycogen (carbohydrate) stores start to deplete. The rule of thumb is 30–60 grams of carbs for every hour you run. Sports drinks have carbs; just be mindful of artificial craziness. Sugar is a fast-acting carb that has its place, but there is such a thing as too much of a good thing.

Common fuel for long runs are energy gels, Shot Bloks, sport beans, and chews. I love Honey Stinger gels with caffeine. These products are engineered to provide carbs, sodium, electrolytes, and sugar. You can find these at running stores and every race expo. During a 13-mile training run I will eat one, and during a marathon I might eat as many as four or five. I think it's a good rule to fuel early and often (consume some calories by drink or food every 20 minutes). Some runners have digestive issues with too much fuel. Find your balance.

This is where your internal monologue comes in. Keep track of how you feel with what you eat and when. Do you feel energized? Sluggish? Running to the bathroom?

MY FAVORITE WAYS TO FUEL FOR LONG RUNS AND MARATHONS

Carb Loading

You should increase your intake of carb-rich foods the days leading up to an endurance event. Your muscles become depleted of glycogen after about 90 minutes of running, and carbohydrate consumption tops up your glycogen stores, equaling more gas in the tank. This is commonly referred to as "carb loading" and more commonly misunderstood as eating bagels topped with pasta topped with donuts.

No. No. No. Yes, you can and should splurge, but do you really want to feel gorged with food to the point of being sluggish on race day? No.

Up to 3–5 days before race day, you should start to add carbs to every meal. The general rule of thumb is adding 3–6 grams of carbs per pound of body weight. Smaller carb-rich meals are friendlier on your digestive system. To make room for the extra carbs, you might need to reduce your fat and protein intake during these meals. Foods with fiber should be consumed judiciously 24 hours before a race.

My perfect pre-race meal is a simple bowl of spaghetti and red sauce or pad thai noodles and usually a glass of red wine. I try to eat dinner the evening before a race by six o'clock, which then gives me at least 12 hours before I have to leave for most races the following morning. As with fueling for during the race, don't try a new dish the day before. Stick with what's tried and true.

On race morning, use whatever worked for your long runs. Again, this goes back to the Rule of Half—half a banana, half a bagel, one piece of toast, or a small bowl of oatmeal. You don't want to overload your body, especially if the race start is less than 2 hours away, to allow for proper digestion. Trust your gut, literally!

DURING MARATHONS I CONSUME THE FOLLOWING FUEL:

- Honey Stinger gels
- Shot Bloks with sodium
- Good ol' H_2O
- Coconut water
- Nuun tablets with water
- Honey—great for low blood sugar
- Clementines
- Raisins
- Dates
- Pretzels
- Plain potato chips
- Frozen grapes—heaven on summer runs

ELEVEN WAYS I FUEL TO DO EPIC SHIT

1. Whatever the name you give to your eating habits (paleo, vegan, gluten-free, anti-inflammatory), let's be real about something: There are no shortcuts. There is no magic pill. Do the work to source the most unprocessed, whole foods you can find and eat them.

2. Alkalinity is a battle worth fighting. Minimizing acid in the body and achieving greater pH balance reduces toxins. Apple cider vinegar (unfiltered, organic like Bragg's) diluted in water or used in raw dishes, such as salads, helps restore alkalinity. It also whitens teeth without artificial teeth-whitening creams or strips.

3. For exercise that is 90 minutes or more, my body requires healthy fats and carbs. My perfect meal 4 hours (enough time to digest to avoid gastric distress during a run) before a long run or race is avocado toast on Ezekiel bread (or any sprouted bread) and an apple with any organic nut butter. If you're sensitive to fiber, couscous with pine nuts, pomegranate, and mint is an amazing carb/fat combo.

4. DIY energy drink with chia seeds and maple syrup. I soak a few tablespoons of chia seeds overnight in almond milk, coconut water, or plain H_2O, and then add some maca for energy and maple syrup for sweetness and a sugar boost. Your taste buds adjust to the simplicity of food. Occasionally, I'll drink Gatorade during a race, but otherwise I don't use the stuff.

5. During ultramarathons, I eat potato chips. No matter how fancy products get, there's nothing that I want more than a bag of plain Lay's at mile 40 of a race. There are times to eat chips. And that's one of them.

6. As a type 1 diabetic, I get a lot of questions about fueling for blood sugar lows. I fuel as most endurance athletes do with fruits, energy gels, and bars. The difference is that I take fuel with me everywhere I go in case of an emergency and I have to fuel super-precisely to carb-count for insulin intake. The balance of insulin/carbs versus anticipated exertion can change based on many factors like hormones, diet, and metabolic rates. It's mad complicated (see page 163 for tips for type 1 diabetics).

7. Chia seeds and quinoa are powerhouse foods. Both pack protein and consistently give me energy to perform. Make a big batch of quinoa on Sunday to eat with meals throughout the week. Add chia seeds to smoothies, salads, stir fry, or oatmeal.

8. Marathoners take in 400–500 calories before mile 20. Hitting the wall is real. If you want to avoid feeling like someone dropped a piano on your back, experiment with fuel that you can consume quickly while running. I have fallen in love with Honey Stinger gels and waffles. Try new things before race day.

9. Ginger comes out of my pores. Ginger shots, ginger tea, and ginger marinades are a daily consumption for me. I love the spice and I believe consistently consuming it has decreased inflammation in my body.

10. Bee pollen helps with lung function. Caution: do NOT use it if you have a bee allergy! If you don't have an allergy, sprinkle some bee pollen in your smoothie or even your water. It really doesn't change the taste.

11. What we think, how we fuel, and what we internalize, both in terms of stimuli and narrative, matter. Food is an intimate relationship. Think about what you're putting in your mouth and don't consume toxic shit!

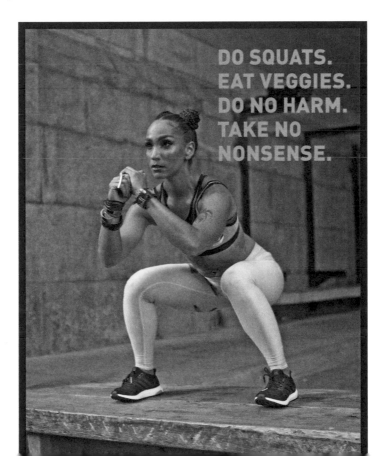

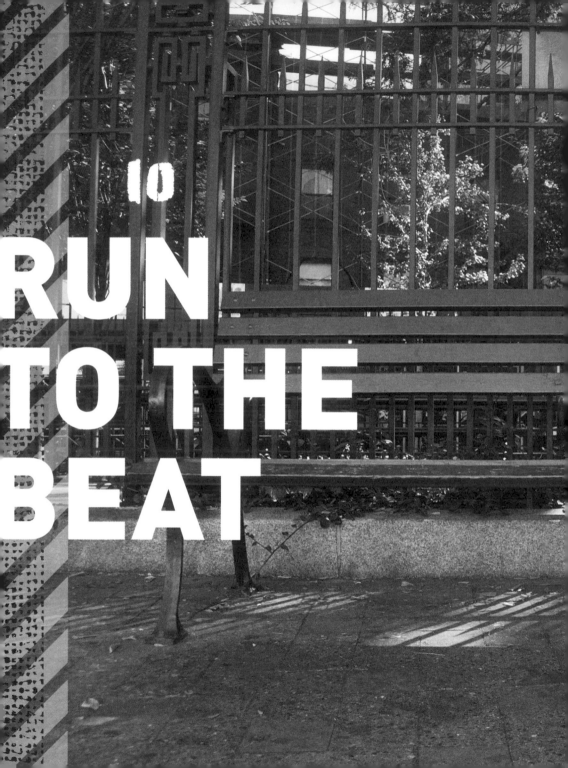

RUN
TO THE
BEAT

"EVERY SUPERHERO NEEDS HIS THEME MUSIC."
—KANYE WEST, "POWER"

RHYTHM IS LIFE AND GREAT BEATS CAN MAKE A RUN.

As a new runner, I couldn't have imagined running a single step without motivational music. I basically woke up every day with Beyoncé as the inspiration to get out there and run. Her music has pushed me through thousands of miles. For real.

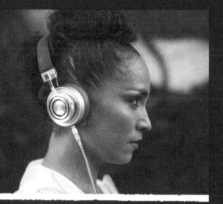

I rarely run with music these days, but music is central to most of my cross-training on the bike, in the gym, and the studio. Most professional runners do not run to music, so they can instead tune in to breath and cadence. Many races also have a no-headphones policy. I subscribe to that now.

FAIR WARNING

There will come a day when your MP3 player dies in the middle of a race (or a rainstorm) and this will teach you the mental dance required to go inside. Until then, this chapter is for you cats who can't run without music.

BEATS PER MINUTE

SONGS HAVE A PARTICULAR NUMBER OF BEATS PER MINUTE; also know as "BPM." The BPM of a song in line with your running cadence married with the right genre can be like seeing a rainbow on a rainy day. Truly, I've had monumental moments on runs when the perfect track comes on. You don't have to run to the beat, but there is a seamless motivation when music is faster than 90 BPMs. The stride of most elite runners is 180 steps per minute, making a playlist of 90+ BPM music hit that sweet spot (90 per leg).

You can figure out the beats of your current music with a cadence app like Cadence Desktop Pro or BPM Assistant. This will analyze your entire library and add the BPM info to the metadata.

Note: this is a higher turnover than most runners naturally use, so it's okay if you're slower than the beat.

EAR CANDY

Here are some jams for the road. Not every song is exactly 90 BPM, but even the slower ones might help to motivate your ass to move. Irrespective of beat, sometimes it's just about the vibe of a track. Some runs will be angry and some will be bubbly. Meet your mind where it is and run it out.

Music preference during a marathon can be a whole different ball game on race day. For my first New York City Marathon, I listened to Ol' Dirty Bastard's "Shimmy Shimmy Ya" on repeat for two hours. Literally. You just don't know what you're going to need in the moment, but also don't be afraid to put the headphones down once in a while.

MY ULTIMATE PLAYLISTS

DIVA INSPIRATION

"Blank Space" by Taylor Swift
"Bad Reputation" by Joan Jett
"Roar" by Katy Perry
"Get Me Bodied" by Beyoncé
"Only Getting Younger" by Elliphant,
  also featuring Skrillex
"FU" by Miley Cyrus
"Do What U Want" by Lady Gaga
"Lighters Up" by Lil' Kim
"Team" by Lorde
"If" by Janet Jackson
"Burn" by Ellie Goulding
"Lady Marmalade" by Christina
  Aguilera, Lil' Kim, Mya, and Pink
"Bitch Better Have My Money"
  by Rihanna
"Kiss with a Fist" by Florence and
  the Machine
"Upgrade U" by Beyoncé
"You Oughta Know" by Alanis Morissette
"Just Fine" by Mary J. Blige
"Work It" by Missy Elliott
"Criminal" by Fiona Apple

HIP-HOP FOREVER

"Hey Ya!" by Outkast
"Izzo (H.O.V.A.)" by Jay-Z
"Get Em High" by Kanye West
"C.R.E.A.M." by Wu-Tang Clan
"Run" by Ghostface Killah
"Rebel Without a Pause"
  by Public Enemy
"I Don't Fuck with You" by Big Sean

"Fu-Gee-La" by Fugees
"Crazy" by Snoop Dogg
"Blood on the Leaves" by Kanye West
"Uptown Funk" by Mark Ronson
"I Wish" by Skee-Lo
"Make Her Say" by Kid Cudi
"Church" by T-Pain
"Hot Boyz" by Missy Elliott
"Sabotage" by Beastie Boys
"The Seed" by the Roots
"I Got 5 on It" by Luniz

ROCK IT OUT

"Can't Stop" by Red Hot Chili Peppers
"Runnin' Down a Dream" by Tom Petty
"Message in a Bottle" by the Police
"Jack & Diane" by John Mellencamp
"Everlasting Light" by the Black Keys
"Song 2" by Blur
"I'm on Fire" by Bruce Springsteen
"The Distance" by Cake
"We Are the Champions" by Queen
"40 Oz to Freedom" by Sublime
"Yellow" by Coldplay

THE ULTIMATE EVERYTHING
PLAYLIST

"Watch Out for This" by Major Lazer
"Recess" by Skrillex and Kill the Noise
"Turn Down for What" by DJ Snake
  and Lil Jon
"Bad Blood" by Taylor Swift
"Unstoppable" by E.S. Posthumus

"Stole the Show" by Kygo
"Freedom" by Pharrell Williams
"I Just Wanna F" by David Guetta
  and Afrojack
"Fatty Boom Boom" by Die Antwoord
"Bang That" by Disclosure
"Burial" by Yogi and Skrillex
"300 Violin Orchestra" by Jorge Quintero
"Lose Yourself" by Eminem
"Dangerous" by David Guetta
"Take a Walk" by Passion Pit
"Shimmy Shimmy Ya" by Ol' Dirty
  Bastard
"Slam" by Onyx

FIGHT SONGS

"Closer" by Nine Inch Nails
"Runnin'" by the Pharcyde
"The Show Goes On" by Lupe Fiasco
"Little Lion Man" by Mumford & Sons
"Paper Planes" by M.I.A.
"Give It Away" by Red Hot Chili Peppers
"Part Time Lover" by Stevie Wonder
"Bap U" by Party Favor
"Indian Summer" by Jai Wolf
"All I Do Is Win" by DJ Khaled
"Lucifer" by Jay Z

STRETCHING JAMS

I'm the worst at taking time to stretch.
Below is a short playlist to listen to as
a cooldown for some post-run TLC.

"Don't Wait" by Mapei
"Superpower" by Beyoncé
"Let It Go" by Michael Franti and
  Spearhead

"Sure Thing" by Miguel
"In the Colors" by Ben Harper
"Mouthful of Diamonds" by Phantogram
"No Diggity" by Chet Faker (cover)
"Fire Meet Gasoline" by Sia
"Home" by Edward Sharpe and
  the Magnetic Zeros
"The Long Road" by Eddie Vedder

NINETIES
HIP-HOP
IS STILL THE
BEST FOR
EVERY MOOD.

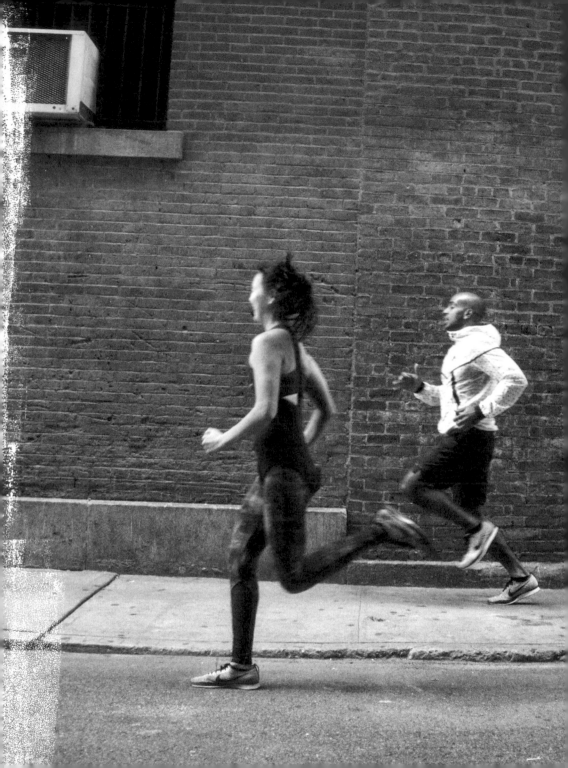

BOOTY
SHAKES
ARE A
GOOD
LIFESTYLE
CHOICE.

LIMITS WERE
MEANT TO BE
TESTED. YOUR
TEST IS YOUR
TESTIMONY.

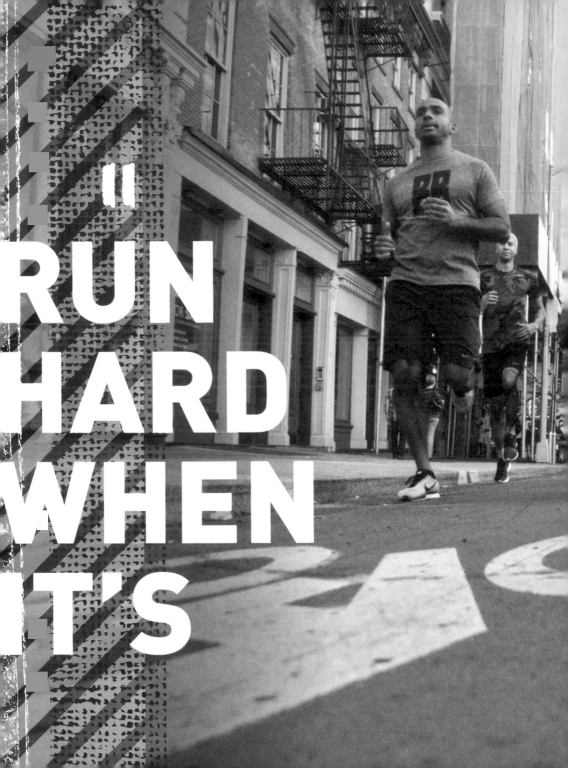

"RUN HARD WHEN IT'S

HARD TO RUN

ENDORPHINS ARE MAGIC.

SUPERHEROES
ARE REAL

GROWING UP I WORSHIPPED the character She-Ra, He-Man's infinitely more badass twin sister. My mom loves telling the story of me dressed up in the She-Ra shield, headpiece, and gold armbands for three Halloweens in a row, and casual Tuesdays. The thing about superheroes that always fascinated me wasn't their extraordinary powers; it was their human fallacies. Even Achilles had a tender spot. For me, my mom is my tender spot. In my "Life as a Movie," the drama gets juicy when something happens to mom.

My mom, a quirky physician born and raised in Cuba, taught me it's better to be bold and weird and to do your own dance, especially when people are watching (she has no rhythm to speak of). She is the type of woman who can light up a room and move mountains without raising her voice. She also has multiple sclerosis (MS), a neurological condition in which an abnormal response of the body's immune system is directed against the central nervous system. The immune system attacks myelin, the fat around nerve fibers, which can cause paralysis, blindness, and a host of other scary conditions.

So what does the superhero do when the world is crumbling, the president is calling, and the landscape is ablaze? She fights.

My mom's MS diagnosis was one of the things that directly fueled my running. I can honestly say I would not be writing this book or have left the legal profession if it weren't for MS. I signed up for my first marathon in 2010 after a breakup, and then I chose to run the New York City Marathon with the National MS Society. Crossing that finish was a game changer. I caught the bug. I realized that running can be transformative. My mom's MS diagnosis was my kryptonite and running was my superpower.

Fast-forward through two New York City Marathons and a number of stair climbs with the MS Society, proudly raising tens of thousands of dollars with the generosity of my tribe. It's 2013 and my mom is having trouble with her eye sight as a result of the villain in this story. As if on cue, I needed some epic shit. I needed to do something when there was nothing to be done. I don't do shackled. I don't do helpless. Enter MS Run the US, a point-to-point cross-country relay from Los Angeles to New York City. In its inaugural year, nobody had heard of this crazy run. Each leg ranged from 150 to 300 miles per runner. At that point, I hadn't run more than 50 miles. It was February and the relay started in March. I had no business signing up to run five marathons in five days just fifteen weeks later, so obviously that's what I did.

My leg of the relay involved five marathons in five days across Utah. The relay ended in New York that August, which would have given me more time to train and more course support, but I couldn't do it. Why? Burning Man. My yearly pilgrimage to run around the desert in sequin booty shorts conflicted with the New Jersey–New York leg. Priorities, babe!

I had never been to Utah. As someone deeply versed in the urban landscape and basically raised by the Wu-Tang Clan, it was funny as hell that I'd be running in nothing but tiny spandex across Mormon country.

Arriving in Las Vegas, I was picked up by filmmaker Tara Darby's camera crew, who would be videotaping my journey for her film in the documentary *Run It Out*. The plan was for MS Run the US founder Ashley Schneider to support me with food and hydration during the run, and we would both stay in the MS Run the US RV during the evenings in between marathons.

On the eve of the first 26.2 leg, I was questioning whether I could actually do this. I had done training involving back-to-back long runs, a few 50-milers, but I did not know if I could complete 130 miles of running. My race was not only public on my social media channels, involving thousands of dollars of donations, but I also had a camera crew following me. This had the potential to be embarrassing as fuck. Mind you, I was completely aware of endurance all-stars who had completed much longer distances, like Scott Jurek, James Lawrence (the "Iron Cowboy"), Dean Karnazes, and now friend Rich Roll, who did five Ironman races in five days. I had perspective cloaked in debilitating doubt.

Day one: 28.5 miles. Milford, Utah. Main Street. The vibes were fantastic. I cut my MS Run the US blazing orange T-shirt into a crop top and canvassed a few thousand feet of elevation. I felt great. At the end of the first 28 miles, I felt strong.

Day two: 55 miles. Thanks to Ashley, Tara, and the crew's encouragement, the second day flew by. I was in such good spirits that I took in the majesty of God's Country (Utah is stunning). It had the potential to make my boyfriend, New York City, jealous.

Day three: 80 miles. My mom and uncle met me on the third day. Spirits were high and emotions were higher. There's something about having people who know you who can lift you as well as gut you to the core. I started to feel the miles, thousands of steps in the right direction, and some hot spots on my feet setting in. Positioned squarely in the middle of promise and potential, I had to go inward.

Day four: 107 miles. By day four, the toenail on my big right toe was starting to rip off. Ashley had to cut the toe boxes off my running shoes to make room for swelling, chafing, ripping, and bleeding. It was so gnarly. Step-by-step rocks embedded in my insoles. One mile felt like ten. My digestive system was a wreck. With zero appetite, Ashley force-fed me liquid protein shakes. I'm certain I was the opposite of appreciative. (Sorry, guys!) I had prepared for physical discomfort when I signed on the dotted line. I knew my legs would ache, my arches would rub raw, and my shoulders would tense. That was the good stuff. The painful moments were in the crevices of my mind. I was feeling defeated and fatigued, but as the day progressed I knew giving up wasn't an option and the pain reinforced my larger goal—finish. At the time, Justin Timberlake had just come out with a new album and all I could do was listen to "Pusher Love Girl" on repeat. For hours. I was slowly losing my shit.

Day five: 131 miles. I absolutely lost it 10 miles from the finish line when the GPS was off and routed me onto a highway. I was on a stretch of road that is the main commercial corridor into Nephi, Utah. As dozens of eighteen-wheelers blazed by, my resolve disintegrated. There's no reasoning with someone who is hanging on by a thread. While I screamed on the side of the road, a rational person could rationalize I'd made it more than 120 miles and I was just steps away. I, however, was brought to my knees and basically crying, crawling, and cursing. Nothing made sense but forward. Ultras are mental. Running was my superpower, but I was doing Jedi mind tricks to take this home.

I finished into the arms of the most insane posse on the planet. I danced under the finish line banner wearing a superhero cape and drinking champagne from the bottle. I couldn't fix my mom. But we weren't going down without a fight. One hundred thirty-one miles across Utah in five days. Sweat is magic.

I run to give the finger to MS. I run because superheroes are real. I run because if you don't try you will never know. Why do you run?

MY RUNNING SUPERHEROES

Florence "Flo-Jo" Griffith Joyner—an American track heroine who evoked sweat with swagger from every pore.

Steve Prefontaine—an American middle and long distance runner, who ran on his own terms and rocked a mustache like no other.

Paula Radcliffe—an Olympic marathon all-star and the current holder of the women's world record in the marathon (2 hours and 15 minutes). So fast, so fierce.

Kara Goucher—an Olympian and fast as hell. But I really love that she has an inner fire that can't be stopped as she fights for every finish and Olympic medal, and she's a badass mom.

CHALLENGE: Make a list of your superheroes. Maybe they're a friend or family member, or maybe they're a fictional character. It doesn't matter, so long as they inspire you.

INSPIRATIONAL SOCIAL MEDIA ACCOUNTS

- Ronda Rousey (@rondarousey)
- Kara Goucher (@karagoucher)
- Allyson Felix (@af85)
- Rich Roll (@richroll)
- Sanya Richards-Ross (@sanyarichiross)
- BridgeRunners (@bridgerunners)
- Dean Karnazes (@ultramarathon)
- Shauna Harrison (@shauna_harrison)
- UNDO-ORDINARY (@undoordinary_)

FITNESS APPS I LOVE

- Tabata Stopwatch Pro—easy interval timer for speed drills and strength work
- Nike+ Training Club—GPS and social push from the community leaderboards
- Charity Miles—run, bike, or walk for charity every mile you log
- Spotify—pick your jams or follow pre-made workout playlists
- Spring Moves—a rhythm-based music app
- Strava Cycling and Running—another GPS tracker and online community to push you
- Headspace—a meditation app

RUNNING BOOKS I LOVE

- *Born to Run* by Christopher McDougall
- *Eat & Run* by Scott Jurek
- *Finding Ultra* by Rich Roll
- *What I Talk About When I Talk About Running* by Haruki Murakami
- *Kings of the Road* by Cameron Stracher

INSPIRATIONAL BOOKS

- *The Power of Now* by Eckhart Tolle
- *A Return to Love* by Marianne Williamson
- *The Fear Project* by Jaimal Yogis
- *Through the Eyes of a Lion* by Levi Lusko

MY FAVORITE TRAINING BIBLES

- *Marathon* by Hal Higdon
- *Meb for Mortals* by Meb Keflezighi
- *Jogging* by William Bowerman
- *Hansons Marathon Method* by Luke Humphrey

GREATEST RUNNING MOVIES EVER

- *Unbroken* (2014)
- *Transcend* (2014)
- *Run for Your Life* (2008)
- *Unbreakable: The Western States 100* (2012)
- *Running the Sahara* (2007)
- *Prefontaine* (1997)
- *Spirit of the Marathon* (2007)
- *Fire on the Track* (1995)

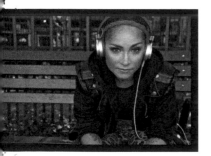

CREW LOVE

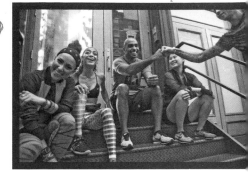

AFTER LAW SCHOOL, I moved back to New York City to practice law at Paul Hastings LLP. As I geared up for my first marathon, I discovered the NYC BridgeRunners. Picture a motley crew that runs because running is life, not a finish line. This world is an ethos-driven existence bonded by sweat and high on endorphins.

BridgeRunners are my family. Founded in 2004 by downtown legend Mike Saes, BridgeRunners have single-handedly taught me that the city is a training partner and courage is contagious. This runners' world is more than fitness or posturing, it's family, because iron sharpens iron mile by mile.

Crews have shown me how to harness the power of community to keep moving. Marathons are a lifestyle and running shoes are the global equalizer. Cities like New York, Paris, and London have unearthed urban running culture. Ranging from ultramarathoners to novice runners, running crew members are uniquely situated at the intersection of sport, culture, and fashion. DJs run with photographers, next to artists and streetwear designers, wherein cultural trends are explored through the lens of athletics. The marriage of the sport and fashion is seamless because, for them, running is a lifestyle.

Social media also fosters the frenetic energy of the running crew culture. Live tweets from training runs create a virtual training environment. From substantive training advice to inspirational messaging, this visual cacophony creates a drumbeat leading up to race day that's echoed in every Instagram snapshot. However, this isn't about posturing. These cats are doing serious distances for the love and the grit of pushing the pulse of the city with their feet. The ethos: train hard, run harder, and play hardest.

Even if you're a solo runner, I encourage you to dabble in group runs. The power of the collective pushes you to demand more of yourself. Whether you are mentoring another runner or they are pushing you to run faster, you will grow. It will reinforce the backbone of why you live this life of sweat.

UNDO-ORDINARY is a fitness collective that I cofounded with Naivasha Colette Thomas. Since its inception in 2013, it's grown into a virtual training platform, a print publication, *UNDO* magazine, and a global community of runners, cyclists, warriors, and badasses. UNDO is about showing how ordinary people can do extraordinary things. Through my running life and the connections born of sweat at UNDO, I know how powerful we are together.

TIPS ON FINDING YOUR RUNNING TRIBE

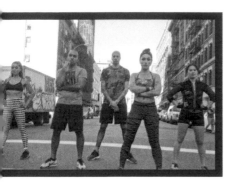

- Put out an APB on social media for runners in your area. Chances are, if you're finding friends of friends through social media to run with, then they are your vibe. If you build it they will come. Clear a path for other runners by running it, boldly.

- Runners go to running stores. Find a local store and talk to them about joining or hosting a group run.

- Sites like Strava, Active.com, and Meetup.com have group run info.

- Train virtually with training partners you've never met. It's surprisingly motivating to see the progress of strangers on apps like Nike+ or MapMyRun. Follow people, track your mileage, and engage. Hashtag campaigns on social media are a solid motivator. Follow @undoordinary_ and @BridgeRunnersNYC. Get inspired. Stay moving.

VISUALIZATION TIP

We're not meant to waste our days. I've been vibe on the simple choice between NOW and LATER. Showing up to the moment is more than a cute self-help sentiment. Your homework right now is to make a public statement of a running goal you will accomplish within **THE NEXT FORTY-EIGHT HOURS**. Is this your first run? Will you sign up for a new race? Do you have a personal record you want to reach? Claim it, because it's already inside you.

YOUR LIFE IS
YOUR MESSAGE.
OWN THE PEN
TO THE STORY
YOU'RE WRITING.
ONE MILE AT A TIME.
IRON SHARPENS IRON.

ACKNOWLEDGMENTS

WELL, DAMN. Lots of people have loved me no matter which hat or suit or spandex I was wearing. It takes a village to handle my brand of crazy. Taylor Swift, we should be friends. Beyoncé, you're my spirit animal. I would pay my taxes to you. Let's go running.

Vasha Thomas, Anna Duren, Sam Turino, Adam Meiras, Casey McGrath, Rachel Ortsman, Candice and Joe Richards, Terrell Pruitt, Stephan Keating, Emily Shen, Sacha Noelle, Linette Guellen, Crystal Joe, Miles Chamley-Watson, Sophia Chang, Jess Lebron, Bangs, Mariah Wilson, Jessica King, Ross Schneiderman, Paula Mitchell, Rich Roll, Mishka Shubaly, Mike Saes, Cedric Hernandez, every single BridgeRunner, global running family in Run Dem, NBRO, PRC, MS Run the US, UNDO, the Participation Agency, Serengeti Animal House, Peloton Cycle, Street Life, Black Rock City, Paul Hastings (my last law firm), Querrey & Harrow (my first law firm), Coach Cane (my first marathon coach), Stephen England (my T1D inspiration), and, of course, Wu-Tang Clan, are just some of the people and groups who got me to NOW.

Twanna Toliver, you are more than an assistant. You could manage everything from the universe to the crevices of my wild brain. Brandi Bowles, agent extraordinaire, thanks for having my back and believing in my message. HarperCollins and my editor Paige Doscher, thanks! This book would literally not be possible without your gorgeous imprint and design team, especially the designer Stephanie Stislow. The imagery in this book is the vision of Ja Tecson and Erin Douglas, and the creative team Renee Sanganoo (makeup) and Encruma Garriques (hair). Thanks for being magic makers.

From aunts and uncles who celebrate me, to cousins who shaped me, to my

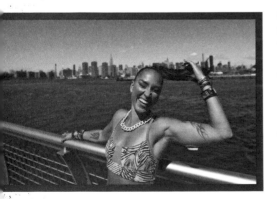

little sister, Margaret, who is infinitely wiser and more inspiring, I come from resilient stock—my family, my original wolf pack, thanks for showing me what it means to roar. Edith, I wouldn't be alive if you didn't watch over me. Dad, I got your creativity, entrepreneurial spirit, legal acumen, and rhythm (thank God).

My north star will always be you, Mom. You, Dr. Carmen Angles, are the queen of queens. You're weird enough to stir the pot and regal enough not to care. There is no me without you.

PHOTOGRAPHY CREDITS

Arzón, Robin: 34, 35, 56, 139 courtesy of Robin Arzón.

Douglas, Erin: 22-23, 28, 45, 54-55, 58-59, 100-101, 109, 111, 119, 120-121, 126-127, 129, 131, 132-133, 152, 170-171, 175, 176-177, 179, 180-181, 186, 187, 188 © 2016 Erin Douglas.

iStock: Page 27, 49, 63, 85, 95, 112-113, 135, 137, 144, 165, 167 courtesy of iStock.

Shutterstock.com: 29 courtesy of Featureflash Photo Agency; 40-41 courtesy of EpicStockMedia.

Tecson, Ja: cover, 2, 8-9, 10, 12, 16, 19, 20-21, 32-33, 36-37, 42-43, 47, 53, 57, 67, 70-71, 74, 76-77, 80, 98, 104-105, 116, 125, 130, 136, 138, 140-141, 143, 146, 150-151, 153, 158-159, 169, 172, 189, 190 © 2016 Ja Tecson.

AUTHOR BIO

AT THE HEIGHT OF HER CORPORATE LAW CAREER, Robin Arzón fearlessly left it all behind to embark on new adventures in the health and wellness space. She soon discovered her passion for coaching athletes.

As a Peloton Cycle senior instructor, she believes that sweat transforms lives. When she's not training for ultramarathons, she serves as a brand ambassador for some of the world's top fitness brands, such as Adidas and formerly Nike, and has successfully become a sought-after partner who connects brands directly to consumers via social media.

As an advocate for the fitness movement Undo Ordinary, she cofounded and serves as editor in chief of the print publication *Undo Magazine*, which combines sweat and fashion. Her life's mission is to redefine, reform, and rethink possibility through movement.

Robin graduated magna cum laude from New York University and Villanova University School of Law. She is a RRCA certified running coach, NASM certified personal trainer, and Schwinn spin instructor. Run with her on Instagram @robinnyc.